The
Whole
Lesbian
Sex Book

A Passionate Guide for All of Us

The Whole Lesbian Sex Book

A PASSIONATE GUIDE FOR ALL OF US

Felice Newman

CLEIS PRESS

Published in the United States by Cleis Press Inc., P.O. Box 14684, San Francisco, California 94114.

Printed in the United States.
Cover design: Scott Idleman
Cover photograph: Phyllis Christopher
Text design: Karen Huff
Logo art: Juana Alicia
First Edition.
10 9 8 7 6 5 4 3 2 1
Illustrations copyright © 1998, 1999 by Fish.

Poems by Sappho are reprinted from *Sappho: A New Translation* by Mary Bernard (University of California Press, 1962), copyright © 1958 by the Regents of the University of California, reprinted with permission. "Rachel Pepper's Tips on Sex During Pregnancy" is excerpted from *The Ultimate Guide to Pregnancy for Lesbians* by Rachel Pepper (Cleis Press, 1999), copyright ©1999 by Rachel Pepper, reprinted with permission. "Fairy Butch's Top Stimulation Tips for Strap-On Sex" is adapted from *The Ultimate Guide to Strap-On Sex* by Karlyn Lotney (Cleis Press, 1999), copyright ©1999 by Karlyn Lotney, reprinted with permission. "Tristan Taormino's Beyond Our Bodies: Emotional and Psychological Aspects of Anal Eroticism" is excerpted from *The Ultimate Guide to Anal Sex for Women* by Tristan Taormino (Cleis Press, 1997), reprinted with permission.

For Frédérique

Acknowledgments

Many thanks to my panel of more than 250 experts—the respondents to my questionnaires without whom this book would not have been possible. Writing from the United States, Canada, United Kingdom, Sweden, Finland, France, Germany, Australia, and New Zealand, they generously shared their experiences, insights, and desires.

I was fortunate to receive the help of many individuals who answered questions, publicized my research and shared the results of their own research, read drafts of chapters, and offered their guidance: Gary Bowen, Cheryl Chase, Constance Clare, Bonnie Faigeles, Suzanna Francis, Nicola Ginzler, Staci Haines, Janet Hardy, Mikaya Heart, Jeanne Marrazzo, Lisa Montanarelli, Cathie Poston, L. E. de Rivaud, Sue Rochman, Cory Silverberg, Shana Sniffen, Tristan Taormino, and San Francisco Sex Information. Many thanks to Karen Huff and Mark Woodworth for design and editing.

Special thanks to David Goldsmith, Terry Rose, Catherine Direen, Barbara Sebastian, and Alesia Kunz, as well as the many other friends who cheered me on!

I am grateful to Susie Bright, Annie Sprinkle, Pat Califia, Tristan Taormino, Carol Queen, Cathy Winks, Anne Semans, and Staci Haines. Their work lit my path.

Finally, my deepest gratitude to my coworkers at Cleis Press, Frédérique Delacoste and Don Weise, who worked twice as hard so that I could write this book.

Contents

ILLUSTRATIONS

Introduction

I HAVE ALWAYS LOVED WOMEN. I've known I was a lesbian for as far back as I can remember. As a little girl, I had dreamy crushes on older girls. My mission was to insinuate myself into the lap of the nearest teenaged girl—and never leave.

I emerged as a tomboy, challenging boys to their own games and resisting the efforts of family members to squeeze me into a female gender that pinched and suffocated and just didn't fit. In high school, I ran with a pack of boys and gazed longingly at the smart girls in my class. To evoke their gaze in return was my highest aspiration.

From my earliest memories, desire for women has fueled my life. I savored small attentions and imagined complicities, "accidental" touches that led to burning kisses, and finally, sex. Sex with women drives my passions like nothing else. I have had sex with many women, and I have been blessed with lovers who offered up their desire with raw courage and lust.

What Makes Me an Expert?

I'm not a social scientist, therapist, or health care worker. I'm a lesbian who has spent many years learning about sex. As publisher of Cleis Press, I've developed and edited books by many of our favorite "sexperts"—from Susie Bright to Annie

Sprinkle. I've trained and served as a hotline volunteer with San Francisco Sex Information. Their 55-hour seminar in human sexuality is the most comprehensive course of its kind. I've spoken on the subject of lesbian sex to all sorts of groups—from teachers earning continuing education credits in Pennsylvania and students at a Christian college in suburban Minnesota to undergrads at the University of California at Berkeley.

But what makes me a lesbian sex expert is that I have devoted myself to erotic exploration. I treat my sex life as an adventure story that builds heat with each episode. I'm curious. Whom will I meet today? What will happen next? I seek abundance. Ample pleasure. Innumerable orgasms. Voluptuous moments bursting with erotic energy. I believe we *all* deserve as much erotic pleasure as life can offer—which is more pleasure really than you or I can conceive of.

I also believe we can teach each other how to have sex. After all, no one else will teach us.

No one ever told us how to be lesbians and bisexual women. No one offered a version of the birds-and-the-bees that spoke to us ("Here is the clitoris. It engorges with blood when aroused and will become erect when caressed…"). No one told us how to ask another girl on a date. Or how to give and receive sexual attention.

I, for one, could have used some guidance. There were years when I wasn't happy with my sex life at all, but I didn't know how to change my circumstances—or even what I might like. Because I hadn't fully explored my own sexual responses, I didn't know what kind of stimulation worked best for me. Instead, I worried that I was missing some vital ingredient, some secret understanding that others possessed.

Years passed. Like many other women, I had bought into the romantic myths about sex. I believed it was my partner's job to "give" me orgasms and to figure out how best to accomplish that. I expected her to read my mind. At the same time, I believed that if I wasn't happy, it was my "fault."

My orgasms felt like appetizers—they left me hungry and restless. Sometimes it seemed to take forever to reach orgasm. I felt demanding and self-centered. I was impossible to please. On some deep level, I didn't think I deserved sexual pleasure.

Like so many women, I wasn't particularly skillful in talking about sex. Although I'm sure we had conversations about sex, I never told my partner of my fears of my own inadequacy. The thought of touching myself or using a dildo or vibrator during partner sex was out of the question. My relationships defined my sexuality. If my lover didn't appreciate sex toys, then the toys stayed hidden in a drawer. Nor was I particularly imaginative in my fantasies—I had pretty fixed ideas about what was and was not OK for a feminist such as myself to get off on.

I felt stuck.

How *On Our Backs* Changed My Life

Really, it was my job at Cleis Press that cracked the ice cap. First, in the late 1980s, Frédérique Delacoste produced *Sex Work: Writings by Women in the Sex Industry,* a book that blew the scalps off feminists on two continents. *Sex Work* made me nervous. If sex workers could stand up to centuries of social stigma to define their own sexualities—some even going so far as to say their work empowered their sex lives—then what the hell was *my* excuse?

Then Susie Bright, editor of *On Our Backs,* tore through what remained of my self-denial. *On Our Backs* appeared on the scene in the mid-eighties. Aimed at the "sexually adventurous lesbian," it was the first lesbian magazine to feature explicit depictions of lesbian sex.

Everyone was talking about *On Our Backs* in those years. Many were shocked by the politically-incorrect implications of lesbians posing for the sexual gaze. Others distanced themselves from the material by critiquing the writing style or production values. Many feminist bookstores refused to carry *On Our Backs* or kept it hidden behind the sales counter.

I stared at the images in those early magazines and read the stories over and over. I wished I felt so comfortable, so powerful, so confident in my erotic life. I suspected, however, that as with all pornography, this was pure hyperbole. No lesbian I knew lived like that, though secretly I wished they did.

But while working with Susie Bright on her collection of columns, *Susie Sexpert's Lesbian Sex World,* I realized that what had seemed incredible to me was no big deal to her. In Susie's world, lesbians engaged in vaginal fisting (which I didn't think was anatomically possible!), had anal sex, visited lesbian strip shows, partied at sex clubs, and generally sparkled with erotic energy.

My imagination lit like a tinder box on a hot afternoon. My complacency and resignation went up in flames, replaced by a broiling dissatisfaction.

I saw the parade passing me by—and I was angry! Enough so to take a hard look at my life and begin to make some changes. I felt awkward and self-conscious. It was like coming out all over again. Thankfully, I found supportive friends and lovers who shared with me their devotion to sexual exploration and personal growth. They prodded me to take risks and applauded my courage. With them, I could delve beyond gossip and nervous tittering to get to the nitty-gritty details of sex. How do you do that? What was that like? How can I do that, too? With their help, I found a language to encompass my own experiences.

I've never looked back. I now can converse easily about sex. I can and do ask for what I need from my partners. I have an active fantasy life—some of my fantasies I act out and some I prefer to remain fantasies. I know what kind of stimulation will best arouse me. I take responsibility for my sex life.

The Whole Lesbian Sex Book

I wrote *The Whole Lesbian Sex Book* so that you would have ample information and encouragement for creating the sex life of your dreams.

Aren't there already lots of books about sex? Yes, and more are published every day. You've probably read horrific treatments of lesbian sex in mainstream sex guides. More recent guides intended for a general audiences, however, do a much better job of representing lesbian sex. Still, we deserve a book of our own.

Often, lesbian sex guides are a bit fuzzy on the actual details of sex. *Sapphistry,* arguably the best of the lesbian how-to books, first appeared in 1979—it's simply dated. Other guides focus on couples, or therapy issues, or brighten your coffee table while telling you very little you didn't already know.

The Whole Lesbian Sex Book is a comprehensive, nonjudgmental guide to lesbian sex—this book won't tell you who you should be or what you should think. You'll find detailed how-to information on sexual techniques, under-standing your own sexual responses, how to have G-spot orgasms, multiple orgasms, and extended orgasms—and much, much more.

During 1999, I developed a series of questionnaires about lesbian sexuality. The questions were very specific, extremely personal, and designed to elicit qualitative rather than quantitative responses. Many of the responses I received were quite explicit. In addition to a lengthy general questionnaire, I devised questionnaires aimed at lesbians and bisexual women who had survived cancer, as well as those who had viral STDs, such as herpes, HPV, hepatitis, and HIV. Posted on the Cleis Press web site, the questionnaires were publicized on Internet mailing lists and in lesbian and gay publications internationally. I received more than 300 responses from 250 respondents (some filled out more than one question-naire)—from the United States, Canada, United Kingdom, Sweden, Finland, France, Germany, Australia, and New Zealand.

Some women wrote pages on one question. Others reported that they had spent several hours on their replies. Some women wrote back with critiques of the questionnaire; in some cases their insights spurred me on to revise my questions. The candor and energy these women put into this project was remarkable. Their responses alone could fill volumes. You'll find them quoted anonymously throughout the book.

I would love to hear from you. Please send me your feedback on this book and your ideas for future editions. If you'd like to be included in research on the next edition of this book, please let me know. You can write to me: WholeLesbian@cleispress.com.

Here's to lesbian sex! May all your desires come true.

Felice Newman
San Francisco
October 1999

chapter one

Welcome

LESBIANS LOVE SEX. We have sex with longtime lovers, crushes, ex-girlfriends, new lovers, fuck buddies, and groups of friends. We even have sex all by ourselves. We have soul-gazing sex, heart-melting sex, and sensual afternoons of bed-flooding sex. We have loud, sweaty, headboard-pounding sex that wakes the neighbors. We have screaming, multiorgasmic sex. We have edgy sex. We have *sex*.

Women have been sexual with other women for as long as human beings have existed. We have loved and desired each other in every culture and in every era. And though since biblical times we've had to read between the lines to discover ourselves in history ("Whither thou goest…"), we continue to delight in the pleasures of sex with women.

You may have been led to believe that lesbians don't have sex (we have caresses) or that we don't have "real" sex (since two women "can do anything a man can—until it comes to that last little detail"[1]). You may have read that women would rather cuddle than fuck (thanks to Dear Abby—or was it Ann Landers?), or that lesbian lovers suffer from Lesbian Bed Death (perhaps a trip to Macy's furniture department is in order?).

Conversely, you may have gotten the message that lesbians are the original connoisseurs of sex. We possess Sapphic secrets refined through centuries of practice, handed down from mentor to novice. Did you know that entire lessons on lesbian eroticism were deleted from the original *Kama Sutra*? If we really do

If you will come

I shall put out

new pillows for

you to rest on.

•

I was so happy

Believe me, I

prayed that that

night might be

doubled for us

•

We shall enjoy it.

As for him who finds

Fault, may silliness

And sorrow take him!

SAPPHO

have such knowledge of female arousal and satisfaction, then we must be erased from history.

Lesbian sex has been envied, outlawed, hidden, packaged, glamorized, erased, pathologized, and obsessed over ever since woman discovered the clitoris. Yet women continue to desire each other.

There are as many ways to have lesbian sex as there are lesbians—*and* bisexual women *and* women who enjoy lifetimes of sex with women without ever once naming their desire.

Think of this book as a resource filled with information, suggestions, tips, and techniques to help you discover a sexuality that works for *you*.

This book is about sex shared between women. Whether you identify as a lesbian or bisexual; butch, femme, or androgynous; traditionally gendered or transgendered— and even if you have just begun to consider the possibility that you, a woman, might desire sex with a woman—this book is for you.

NOTES:
1. Dr. David Reuben, M.D., *Everything You Always Wanted to Know About Sex (but Were Afraid to Ask)*, 2nd ed. (HarperCollins, 1999), 163. In the original 1969 edition, the quote was "one vagina plus one vagina equals zero."

chapter two

Desire and Fantasy

*Fantasies, like dreams or myths, are ways we talk to ourselves
about our most profound truths.—*DOSSIE EASTON [1]

WHAT DO LESBIANS AND BISEXUAL WOMEN DESIRE FROM OUR WOMEN LOVERS?
Well, just about everything you can imagine—and more! We want the fullness of
a woman's sex in our hands and our mouths and between our legs. We want to
drink our own juices from her fingers. We want to feel her breasts and taste her
nipples.

We desire bountiful, luscious, mind-altering moments of pleasure. We nurture dreams we would never make real and dreams we would leap at the chance
to fulfill—the hungry gaze of a stranger, the astonishment of a lover revealed in
orgasm, bodies like and unlike our own, discovery, transformation, exposure,
secrecy, need yielding to force, and need yielding to need. And then—with an
unexpected touch, a glance of skin in a spill of light, humidity flavored by sex—
we drown in memory.

What do *you* desire sexually? Do you want the same things today that you
wanted ten years ago? One year ago? Last week? What turned you on at 12 may
have seemed quite silly at 16, and what you liked at 16 may evoke little but
nostalgia now. So why would you think that what heats you up now will suffice
for the rest of your active sex life?

The inner voice of Eros is arbitrary, bizarre, impeccably honest, bountiful, and so powerful as to be cruel. It takes courage to hear its demands and follow them.

PAT CALIFIA

What desires do you allow yourself? Is it OK for a dyke to fantasize about sex with a man? Sex *as* a man? Is it OK for a survivor of violence to masturbate to rape fantasies? Are you betraying your partner if you fantasize about other people? Her best friend, for instance?

Desire is a slippery beast. What actually stirs you to passion may bear little resemblance to what you *say* you want. Or what you think you *should* want. You may have no idea why a particular scenario makes your heart race. You need not understand or even approve of your desires. You can keep up with the latest theories in the popular press, but you'll probably never really know why you desire women, or men, or both.

Your desires are uniquely yours. You have your own constellation of fantasies, needs, and turn-ons, plus your own history of sexual attractions and experiences. Your desires reveal who you are, where you came from, what's important to you, what you yearn for, and what you fear. No good will come from attempting to mold your desire into something that looks like everyone else's. Indeed, that's the surest route to ending up with no desire at all. The key to developing a sexuality that will challenge and delight you is to bless every crazy twist and turn of your erotic imagination.

I am a huge exhibitionist.
I wear transparent, lacy, laced-up things
with bits of flesh exposed. Slits in my gowns
that go up to here. I get a lot of attention....

What's Your Fetish?

Are you turned on by six-inch stilettos? What about engineer's boots polished to gleaming obsidian? Does an exquisite Victorian corset make your blood pound? Perhaps you work up a sweat over leather, lace, latex, rubber, or fur?

A fetish is an erotic attachment to an ordinarily nonsexual activity, inanimate object, or body part. What qualifies as a fetish is a matter of opinion. According to Freud, a fetish "bears some relation to the normal sexual object but is entirely unsuited to serve the normal sexual aim"—heterosexual procreative sex was what Freud had in mind.[2] By that definition, you could argue that *all* lesbians and bisexual women are fetishists, since we share an interest in erotic practices outside Freud's "normal sexual aim."

What may have seemed fetishistic to Sigmund Freud may be a staple of your erotic fare, and what seems exotic to you may be someone else's sexual routine. Many people think of unusual sexual activities as "kinky" or fetishistic simply because they're unfamiliar. (Conversely, Pat Califia quips that much truly fetishistic behavior passes as normal because it has become so widespread no one notices it anymore. The heterosexual American male attachment to big breasts comes to mind.[3])

Originally, a fetish was an object believed to have magical powers—for example, a small carved figure of an animal thought to heal or protect its owner. A fetish object was "regarded with awe…as the embodiment of a potent spirit."[4] Thus a strap-on dildo can be viewed as a fetish, in the classic sense of an object invested with erotic desire and power. Many butches and female-to-male transsexuals (FTMs) would disagree with that label, however; for them, wearing a strap-on dildo represents an expression of their deeply held gender identity.

Fetishes can develop ritualistically around necessities like safer-sex practices. Snap on a latex glove in certain lesbian circles and watch the heads turn. Clothing reserved for erotic use is seen as fetishistic. Often fetish gear is too revealing to wear on the street—for instance, a body suit with a cut-out crotch. But not always—sometimes context creates the eroticism. A man who walks into a sex club attired in a business suit will seem out of place, and he may be asked to leave. A dyke in a suit and tie can breeze past the "Fetish Gear Required" sign, knowing she'll be viewed as delightfully kinky. That same cross-dressing dyke may pass so well on the street that no one blinks an eye. Likewise, patent leather mary janes with little lacy anklets under a Catholic-school-girl plaid skirt won't raise an eyebrow—until worn by an adult woman whose tight blouse reveals abundant cleavage.

Fetishes involving costume are perhaps the most widely known and practiced. Leather chaps, revealing lingerie, severe corsets, latex dresses, rubber hoods, and chain-mail chest harnesses are popular items of fetish gear. Many women have uniform fetishes and go to considerable effort to acquire authentic dress of soldiers, sailors, and cops—right down to the billy club. Uniform fetishists may or may not be exhibitionists.

Many women enjoy erotic practices such as spanking, bondage, and water sports (also called piss play or golden showers). A hot stream of urine splashing from one woman's body onto another's is an intense turn-on to many women. (To play safe, keep urine away from broken skin and the eyes and mouth.)

Body modification, such as tattoos, piercings, scarification, and cuttings, holds deep significance for many. Some eroticize the experience of getting (or giving) a body modification; others are more interested in the result. You can think of genital shaving as a temporary body modification. The ritual of shaving one's own genital area can heighten the anticipation of a hot date. Shaving a partner's genitals can make for an exciting encounter. See "Genital Shaving" in Chapter 8, "Clitoral Play."

Whether you call your erotic interest a fetish or simply a turn-on is up to you. The point is that you feel free to develop your interests. Lesbians and bisexual

Once, we had sex in an airplane.
We pulled the blanket up and she put
her fingers in my cunt. I was coming quietly,
high above New Orleans.

women engage in many different fetish practices, more than could possibly be listed here. You can find organizations, books, magazines, web sites, and online discussion groups devoted to a particular fetish (see "Resources").

Run Wild

But what if you just don't know what you *want?* Many women come to sex with a frustrating sense of vagueness. Sure, your clit leaps to meet your partner's desire—but on your own, you don't know what you want. Even if you have a pretty good idea of what heats you up, embarrassment may keep you from fulfilling those desires. Worse yet, that cold stone of shame caught in your gut says you're wrong no matter *what* you want. Or, you may despair over ever finding a partner whose desires will match yours. You haven't met a likely candidate yet—so why bother? Like unpicked fruit, your fantasies might just as well wither and die on the vine.

You may not have found much support for your sexual desires. Our sexual needs are so often ignored, politicized, or repackaged for someone else's pleasure. The good news is that there *is* support for you to nurture your desires—though finding it will take some creativity (and courage) on your part. (This book lists hundreds of helpful resources, for instance!)

Allow your imagination to run wild. Suspend judgment. Desires are not social contracts. You don't have to act out your fantasies—unless you want to! Who cares whether your fantasies would rate high marks for cinematography or plausibility? The goal here is to find out what makes your juices run. Forget the political ramifications of your desires. (Don't feel guilty about that rape fantasy. Volunteer an extra shift on the crisis hotline.)

My legs become swan's wings,
and I see the wings lifting up out of the water.

Make Your Dreams Come True

The paradox, of course, is that to build sexual self-esteem you have to act as if you already have it. So, here are some suggestions to start you out:

What Do You Want?

- Listen to your gut—actually, listen to your cunt! Desire is in your body. What makes your clit throb?
- Look to your fantasy life. What images pop into your mind during those unguarded moments on waking—or just before orgasm? Your own erotic imagination is a ripe resource for discovering your desires.
- Brainstorm. Grab pencil and paper and make three lists: (1) every sexual activity you've experienced; (2) every sexual activity you've heard about and think you might like to try; (3) every sexual scenario you've ever fantasized. Add to your lists as you come up with new ideas. Don't worry about whether you'll actually do these things—just write them down. (I tried this exercise with a group of women; it's amazing how other people's turn-ons can give you ideas.) See "Erotic Play" later in this chapter.
- Keep a journal of your own erotic journey. You'll be glad to have a record of your own sexual evolution. Who knows? You may end up in an erotica anthology someday!
- Read erotica. Collections of erotic short stories, such as the annual *Best Lesbian Erotica* series, are great resources for mining the erotic imaginations of 20 or more creative, articulate authors each year.
- Read sex guides. You'll find informative, detailed descriptions of things others do or like or desire.
- Rent a video. Porn is a great source for erotic inspiration.

Do Yourself a Favor

- Don't feel as if you'll ever have the sex life of your dreams? Then grant yourself one erotic pleasure every day—even a small one. Buy the current issue of *On Our Backs*, the lesbian sex magazine. Try out your new pocket rocket vibrator at lunch time. Imagine sex with that new receptionist at the gyne's office: "First, I'll get her into the exam room, then I'll put her in the stirrups...."

- "Forbid yourself nothing" is the rallying cry at Stormy Leather, a San Francisco fetish boutique. The creators of all those scrumptious fashion designs in latex and leather would certainly know! New clothes, a new sex toy, a fresh haircut, that tattoo or piercing you've always dreamed of.... Indulge yourself.

- Fantasize about things that delight you, things that frighten you, and things that powerfully turn you on. You can even fantasize about things that you find revolting. It's fine to fantasize about people other than your lover or to fantasize outside your gender preference. You can fantasize about things you may not want to do. You can even have "nonconsensual" sex in your fantasies.

- Declare a day of pleasure without guilt. For one day, imagine the unimaginable.

Find Support

- Find friends who will encourage you in your self-explorations.
- Ask for support. Be specific: "I want to be more vocal about my desires. How did you get over your shyness?"
- Sign on to a sexuality-related Internet discussion group (see "Resources"). Ask the list members how they came to revel in their most challenging desires. (They'll be glad you sparked such a fascinating conversation!) E-mail mailing list subscriptions are free, and many public libraries now provide free Internet access.
- Ask an expert. You may be surprised to learn that many well-known sex-positive authors and artists started out just like you. They may have been just as shy as you. They may have struggled just as painfully for self-acceptance. That's why they've dedicated themselves to making the road easier for you! Check out the "Bibliography" for work by Susie Bright, Loren Cameron, Pat Califia, Kate Bornstein, Carol Queen, and many more.
- Ask your friends to tell you their hottest fantasies. Tell them yours.

Erotic Play

Lesbians and bisexual women enjoy many different erotic activities and turn-ons.
Not all of us share all of these turn-ons—in fact, we may not have even heard of some of them!
(See the "Index" to find discussion of terms you may be unfamiliar with.)

anal penetration

blindfolds

blood play

bondage

breast whipping

breath control

caning

caressing

cocksucking (detatchable or
    not)

consensual humiliation

cracking a whip

cross-dressing

cuddling

cunnilingus

cybersex

dancing

deep penetration

dildos

dominance/submission

double penetration

dressing slutty

dripping hot wax

enemas

exhibitionism

fantasizing

finger fucking

fisting

flirting

frottage

fucking

gazing into a lover's eyes

genderplay

getting a tattoo

golden showers

group sex

hair pulling

holding hands

hugging

ice cubes on her belly

kissing

kneeling

knife play

lacing up her corset

lap dancing

leather, rubber, or latex
    clothing

licking her feet

making videos

massage with sensual oils

Master/slave role-play

masturbating with a vibrator

negotiating sex

nibbling ears and neck

nipple clamps or clothespins

orgasm

outdoor sex

over-the-knee spanking

packing a dildo in your 501s

paying for sex

phone sex

playing with sex toys

polishing boots

putting on a condom

putting on makeup

rape scenes

reading erotica

reapplying your lipstick

renting porn

rimming

role-play

seduction

sensory deprivation

sex in secret

shaving

snapping on a glove

strap-on sex

stripping

sucking her labia

sucking her nipples

talking dirty

tickling with feathers

tribadism

triple penetration

using Saran wrap

voyeurism

wearing a butt plug

wrestling

writing in a journal about sex

Nurture Your Libido

Libido is sexual energy in its purest state—that feeling of *wanting*, regardless of *what* you want. Libido isn't about how you look, the size of your toy chest, or who wants (or doesn't want) to have sex with you. Your libido is your erotic life force, an intrinsic part of who you are. While you may identify many sources of your fantasies, *you* are the source of your desires.

Think of libido as something you practice—like singing, painting, or dancing. Not only do you gain sexual skills with practice, but you find that your capacity for sexual energy (and even sensation) expands. There are many ways to "exercise" your libido: masturbating, fantasizing, having sex with a partner, watching others having sex, viewing porn, reading erotica, talking about sex, planning for sex, and reading sex guides like this one.

Falling in love, of course, is the universal libido enhancer. Coming out can gear up your sex drive (and you can come out over and over, as you discover new ways to channel your erotic energy). Improved body image, self-esteem, and general health will make room for renewed sexual energy. Anything that expands what you allow yourself sexually will pump up your sexual energy.

Libido evolves over the course of a lifetime, ebbing and flowing in a rhythm that's natural for you. Many women notice they feel particularly sexual just before or during their menstrual period. While hormones certainly affect libido, they're not solely responsible for the dips and peaks in your sex drive. After all, many postmenopausal women have hot sex lives, and many premenopausal women notice no connections between their menstrual cycles and their desire for sex.

Pregnancy is well known to affect libido. For many women, desire diminishes during pregnancy. Writes Rachel Pepper: "If you are one of those lucky women who feel more sexual during pregnancy or manage to maintain your normal sexual prowess, more power to you! However, for the vast majority…sexual desire tends to dip."[5]

Stress can affect libido. Depression, of course, dulls all life energy. Recovery from sexual abuse, addiction, or codependency can wreak havoc on one's sense of oneself as a sexual being. Facing a serious illness such as cancer—and enduring the treatments for it—will affect libido. Severe weight gain or loss will affect sex drive.

Basically, anything that challenges body image or self-esteem can affect your sexual energy.

Sex + Intimacy

"Healthy eroticism does not avoid problems; it works with and transforms them," writes Jack Morin, in *The Erotic Mind: Unlocking the Inner Sources of Sexual Passion and Fulfillment*. Morin articulates an equation we all can understand: *attraction + obstacles = excitement.*[7] The forbidden object of desire—whether a person, a fantasy, or a taboo activity—gets us hot like nothing else.

What happens when you take away the obstacle? Sometimes excitement withers, as in the case of longtime lovers whose desire has waned. No longer risking new levels of intimacy, no longer challenged by the process of discovering themselves sexually, they utter the sad lament "The thrill is gone!" Sometimes familiarity breeds not contempt, but boredom.

It's rare that a couple's desire for one another will remain constant through the years. We've all

15 Ways to Heat Up Your Marriage

The mystery is gone, you say? Well, perhaps the challenge of the chase is over, but what's more challenging than sustaining sexual intensity with the woman whose toothbrush drips dry each morning next to yours? Here are some suggestions to help wake up your sex life:

1. Indulge…*yourself!* Read erotica, watch porn, masturbate. Fantasize. Undress the pretty girls on the bus. Fixate on that FedEx woman who dashes into your office every morning. Like any other talent, without exercise your libido will atrophy.

2. Take responsibility for yourself. Remember when your sexuality was yours alone— and not marital property? Regardless of your marriage vows, your girlfriend is not in charge of your inner life or who you dream about when you pleasure yourself.

3. Take a vacation together. Send the kids to your favorite PFLAG mom. Leave town. Don't take your dog.

4. Get out of the bedroom. Have sex in the kitchen. Or the back seat of your old Chevy. Go to a sex club.

5. Take your girlfriend sex-toy shopping— online or at your favorite sex-toy boutique. Giggle. Be embarrassed together. Not interested in toys? Rent a video instead.

6. Use lube. Lots of lube. When you were dating, you probably left wet spots on restaurant seats. Since the first flush of love has faded, your arousal level has tamed and your juices aren't flowing at

quite the same rate. Put some lube on your fingers before you touch your sweetie's clit. The increased wetness will lead to increased sensitivity and increased turn-on. Do the same for yourself when you masturbate.

7. Stop being lazy about sex. You've probably been getting each other off the same way for years. You touch her; she touches you. You lick her; she licks you. Your fist goes in her vagina; her didlo goes in your anus. Over and over, year after year. Even a great program loses something in reruns. Next time you hop in the sack, declare your usual sexual activities off limits. Unplug that tired old toy—or get a new one.

8. Similarly, if your sex play is exclusively genitally focused, try something different. Take turns giving each other full-body massages. Try this exercise from *The Survivor's Guide to Sex:* Sit facing each other on the bed. Breathe together. Run your fingers along her face and neck. Appreciate her. Describe what you're seeing and feeling. Take turns. [6]

9. Switch. After all these years of being the top, have you secretly wanted to throw your heels in the air? Or have you nurtured a secret fantasy of giving your aggressive girlfriend a taste of her own medicine? 'Fess up, now!

10. Sure, your best friend can recite your marital disappointments blow for blow. But have you talked with your partner about your sexual frustrations? Are you afraid that if you tell her your complaints, she'll tell you hers, and you'll realize you're not so happy after all, and soon you'll be down $90 a week for couple's counseling—forget that trip to London—and besides, you'll just break up anyway…. Whew! Talk to your partner; tell her your erotic hopes and dreams.

11. Speak in positives; don't dump. Unless you've negotiated a humiliation scene, telling your lover of six years that she bores you is not likely to improve your sex life! Remind her how much you love her. Tell her you'd like to have the sex life of your dreams—with her. Be specific. Know what you want and ask for it. (See Chapter 6, "Communication and Finding Sex Partners," for hints.)

12. Don't assume you know what she likes, either. Ask.

13. Be blissfully wedded…novices. Pick a sexual activity neither of you has ever done—and do it. Never played with anal beads? Rope bondage? Attended a live erotic performance? Have you thought of cross-dressing?

14. Find a role model. Whether in a self-help book or on your dyke rugby team, find someone who's in an intimate relationship and has hot sex. Get details!

15. Face your demons. Bet this isn't the first time your desire has fizzled out on a lover. If so, you're not alone! Many people find intimate relationships daunting. Why does closeness snuff out your desire? Why do you want to bolt before the ink is dry on the rental agreement? Finding the answers will require some soul searching, and maybe some help. Do you want an intimate sex life—really? You may have to work very hard to achieve that, but the results can pay off, bigtime.

experienced the intense sexual high of falling in love and then the inevitable cooling-out. Of course, "cooling-out" doesn't mean giving up sex. But maintaining a charged sex life with a long-term partner requires attention.

The most common sexual complaint among long-term partners is "desire discrepancy." One partner wants *more* sex than the other, or one partner wants *different* sex than the other. This can be very threatening to partners in a valued relationship. It's tempting to simply ignore the problem—but that won't help. Faced with desire discrepancy, many people opt for a new partner—or give up on sex. As Morin writes in *The Erotic Mind*, reconciling desire discrepancy can be more subtle than that. For instance, you could keep the lover but change the sex. Morin encourages a process of self-exploration and discovery to help you find out what really makes your libido cook.

Many self-help books are available to help solve the problem of desire discrepancy among couples. See the "Bibliography" for suggestions.

Fantasy

Fantasies are great ways to find out what you want sexually. You can try on new sexual activities, styles, and genders in your fantasies. You don't have to be too literal in interpreting your fantasy. That six-woman gang bang you revisit each night before sleep isn't proof of a death wish or a deep need to be defiled. It may just be that you want to give up control, have group sex, or be overwhelmed by your partner's desire for you.

Here are some fantasy classics:

- *Anonymous sex.* "I'm in a crowded bar. We make eye contact and go off to a dark corner. I lift her skirt...." Hotel cocktail lounges are often the settings for fantasies involving sex with strangers (all those bedrooms just an elevator ride away...). The rough-trade version of this fantasy can be set in the subway, an alley, or the back room of a gay bar. Money exchange provides an extra twist.
- *Romance.* We fantasize about falling in love, with soulful gazes and heart-shattering desire. "It's summer and the mangos are ripe. We're lying in bed with the fan on, feeding each other and licking off the stickiness...."

- *Cross-orientation.* Many people change sexual orientation in their fantasies. Lesbians can and do get off to fantasies of sex with men. In our fantasies, we can be straight girls or dykes, dominant or submissive; we can be femmes having sex with men or butch dykes having group sex with bodybuilders at a gay sex club.
- *Gender shifts.* "I pull out my dick (in the fantasy it's real) and start beating off. She reaches down and takes the head of my dick in her mouth and starts sucking really slowly, finally taking it all the way down her throat." In your dreams you can change gender a dozen times in one night. You can also try out sex in the gender that's true for you.
- *Dominance.* Many of us fantasize having a partner on her (or his) knees, begging for mercy, for attention, for release, for a spanking, or for an orgasm.
- *Submission.* "I need someone to take control," wrote one woman, echoing a common theme. "In my 37 years I have not had that kind of sex, but have always dreamed of it."
- *Discipline.* "I am bent over the teacher's desk with no panties on, getting spanked for some infraction in front of the entire class—boys and girls. Sometimes the teacher designates a boy to fuck me after the spanking."
- *Age play.* Hot scenes can come from role-playing in which adult partners adopt age-based (and gender-based) power roles. Daddy/girl, Daddy/boy, Mommy/girl, Mommy/boy roles are popular forms of age play.
- *Exhibitionism.* Up on the roof, under the boardwalk, or in the back seat of a taxi, public sex can be a big turn-on. Wearing revealing clothing and arranging to be "caught" masturbating are also common themes.
- *Famous partners.* Sigourney Weaver, David Bowie, Amelie Mauresmo, Joan Jett, Leonardo DiCaprio...and, as one lesbian wrote, "A Tilly sandwich— Jennifer Tilly and her sister Meg Tilly."
- *Threesomes.* "I'm going down on a woman and a man is fucking me from behind."
- *Initiation rites.* "Taking" a virgin, teaching a novice new tricks, bringing out a straight woman. "Sometimes I fantasize that I'm am a virgin...."

- *Molestation.* "I want to be a little girl selling Girl Scout cookies. I ring a bell and a very handsome man answers the door with only a towel wrapped around his waist...."
- *Role-play.* "In my favorite fantasy, I'm the ship's wench on a co-ed pirate vessel. I'm tied spread-eagle to a giant roulette wheel in a dark room deep in the hull of the ship."
- *Rape.* "I'm forcing another femme to have sex—tying her up and ass-fucking her." The debate about rape fantasies usually focuses on the woman-as-victim. But what about women who fantasize being the rapist?
- *Edge play.* Water sports, blood play, scarification, severe sadomasochism (S/M).
- *Taboo sex.* Vampire play, bestiality (sex with animals), necrophila (sex with the dead).

Suggested Web Links:

THE WOMB
   womb.wwdc.com/fetish.html
A DYKE'S WORLD
   Wild Women Dreamin' Wet—Lesbian erotic stories
   www.dykesworld.de

NOTES

1. Dossie Easton, San Francisco Sex Information continuing education workshop, San Francisco, March 22, 1999.

2. Sigmund Freud, "Three Essays on Sexuality," in the *Standard Edition of The Complete Psychological Works*, vol. 7 (Hogarth Press, 1953). As quoted in *The Deviant's Dictionary*, online encyclopedic dictionary of S/M-related terms, 1997. www.queernet.org/deviant

3. Pat Califia, *Public Sex: The Culture of Radical Sex* (Cleis Press, 1994), 172. She continues, "However, much fetishism probably passes as 'normal' (nonfetishist) sexuality because the required cue is so common and easy to obtain that no one notices how necessary they are."

4. *Webster's Unabridged Encyclopedic Dictionary* (1989 edition), as quoted in alt.sex.fetish.fashion, 1996. See www.sexuality.org/l/fetish/fashion.html

5. Rachel Pepper, *The Ultimate Guide to Pregnancy for Lesbians* (Cleis Press, 1999), 126.

6. Staci Haines, *The Survivor's Guide to Sex* (Cleis Press, 1999), 237.

7. Jack Morin, *The Erotic Mind: Unlocking the Inner Sources of Sexual Passion and Fulfillment* (HarperPerennial, 1996), 50.

SOURCE OF QUOTE

Pat Califia, *Public Sex: The Culture of Radical Sex* (Cleis Press, 1994), 113–14.

chapter three

Anatomy and Sexual Response

My pussy is a very lovely, shorn, shapely, and soft thing.

LET'S BEGIN WITH A TOUR OF YOUR SEXUAL ANATOMY. Regardless of how you relate to your body—whether you're comfortable being female, love your genitals, hate your genitals, or feel your body is the perfect expression of who you are—your sex life will be enhanced by understanding what's going on down there.

Anatomy

The official term for the female genitalia is *vulva*. Some of us prefer *pussy, cunt,* and other names. Our genitals include the clitoris, labia, and vagina. The fleshy area over the pubic bone is called the mons. Our perineum, anus, and breasts can also be quite sensitive to sexual stimulation.

Truth is, there are women who don't know where or what their clit is—and there are even lesbians who have never held open their labia and looked at themselves. Why? Well, for starters, we're not exactly encouraged to look at our genitals. If only we were presented mirrors, speculums, and Annie Sprinkle videos with those first packages of sanitary pads or tampons.... (As far as I'm concerned, sex ed would best be team-taught by Betty Dodson and Annie Sprinkle, and not your boring, uptight 5th grade science teacher. *A New View of a Woman's Body, Our Bodies Ourselves for the New Century,* and *Femalia* should be required reading. For both girls *and* boys. "*Can you spell c-l-i-t-o-r-i-s? No diploma for you, Johnny!*")

Add to the lack of basic information about our bodies the complicated relationship many lesbians have to gender. Some of us experienced considerable pressure to look and act "feminine"—when we didn't feel feminine inside. Others of us found that our natural femininity made our sexual choice suspect—and, because we looked, dressed, walked, and talked like "normal" women, we felt invisible as lesbians. As a preteen, you may have felt you failed at being the little girl your parents had so wanted. That made it hard to relate to the anatomy diagrams in the package insert that came with your first box of tampons.

Finally, one out of three girls is sexually abused before reaching adulthood. Our sexuality was the site of our pain. No wonder so many of us are shut down, having only a vague notion of what's going on between our legs.

So, let's take a little tour of our genitials.

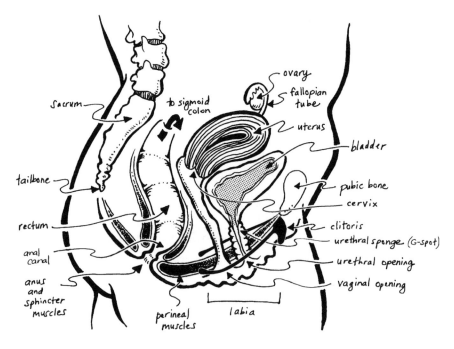

ILLUSTRATION 1. FEMALE ANATOMY

Clitoris

The clitoris is the most sensitive spot in your genital area. If you draw your finger up from your vaginal opening in one long stroke, you'll find your clit at the top of the vulva. (If you like, visualize a clock, with your vaginal opening at six o'clock and your clit at midnight.)

How big is a clitoris? Clits come in a wide variety of sizes, shapes, colors, and sensitivities. Clits can be so tiny you can hardly find them or as big as the first joint of your thumb. Female-to-male transsexuals taking testosterone can develop clits as large as three inches long.

The body of the clitoris is made up of the glans (or head), the hood, and the shaft. The glans is the most sensitive part of the clit, analogous to the head of a penis—only far richer in nerve endings and thus more sensitive. Your clitoral hood drapes your glans and keeps it moist and sensitive—still, touching your unaroused or unlubricated clitoral glans can be irritating or even painful. If you gently hold your clit between your thumb and forefinger, you can feel the shaft.

Hardly the little "nub" described in mainstream sex guides and anatomy texts, the clitoris is a complex structure of erectile tissue, much of which surrounds the urethra—no surprise to women who experience ejaculation with orgasm. Current research conducted by Helen E. O'Connell of the Royal Melbourne Hospital in Australia redefines the clitoris as consisting of the body (glans, hood, and shaft), the crura, and the bulbs: "...the external tip of the clitoris, or glans, connects on the inside to a pyramid-shaped mass of erectile tissue, far larger than previously described."[1]

The crura (or legs) of the clitoris "flare backwards into the body," extending into the vaginal wall on either side of the urethra. (Think of a wishbone, with the clitoral glans in the middle and the crura as the legs.) Called the "vestibule bulbs" in traditional anatomy texts because they sit on either side of the vaginal opening, the "clitoral bulbs" (so named by O'Connell) are analogous to the bulb of erectile tissue at the root of a penis, though, O'Connell says, "the bulbs are more prominent in females." The clitoris, she concludes, is far larger than the tiny structure depicted in conventional anatomy texts.

Why does any of this matter? Well, if you think of your clitoris as an extensive sexual organ—one that protrudes at the top of your vulva, reaches down to flank the vaginal opening, extends into the vagina, and cradles the urethra—your concept of touching your clit just might take on new dimensions!

Labia

The labia majora are the large outer lips of your vulva. These are what some women call their pussy lips. They're usually covered with hair, and the skin is the same texture and color as the rest of you. Among women who shave their genitals, this is the area that's most commonly shorn. The labia minora are next as we move inward. These are asymmetrical, delicate folds of tissue with the same texture as mucous membrane. Generally hairless, they become quite slippery during sex. Some women's inner labia are long, extending outside the labia majora; others are smaller and tucked away inside the labia majora.

Vagina

The opening of the vagina sits below the clit and urethral opening, and above the perineum and anus. The vagina is made up of very elastic tissue that opens up and expands during arousal (and childbirth, of course). When not aroused, the walls of the vagina touch—we do *not* have a big "hole" in there.

The outer third of the vagina contains the most nerve endings, and most women find it to be more sensitive than the deeper areas of the vagina. The opening and G-spot are the most responsive to the subtleties of movement and touch; the deeper areas are more responsive to the pressure of thrusting. The vagina ends in the cervix, the knob-like opening to the uterus through which menstrual blood passes. Some women love to have their cervix pounded; others hate it. Be careful not to bruise or abrade your cervix.

The vagina isn't a passive receptacle. The opening of the vagina is quite muscular. Surrounded by the pelvic muscles, the vagina will contract with pleasure, gripping a finger, dildo, or hand.

G-Spot

The G-spot is named for Ernst Grafenberg, an ob-gyn—but let's think of it as the girl spot, after which a famous roving lesbian club in San Francisco was named. (Their slogan: *The G-Spot—if you can't find it, you can't come!*)

The G-spot isn't a magic button, but rather an area of tissue that feels a bit rougher in texture than the rest of the vagina walls. You can find your G-spot by inserting a finger into your vagina and making a "come hither" motion toward the front wall of the vagina. The G-spot is actually the urethral sponge, an area of tissue surrounding the urethra, which runs along the front wall of your vagina carrying urine from the bladder to the urethral opening. (The urethral opening is located below your clit, just above your vagina.)

Some women ejaculate with G-spot stimulation; some ejaculate with clitoral stimulation. Some like G-spot stimulation, but don't ejaculate. And others find G-spot stimulation too intense to be pleasurable.

Perineum

Between your vagina and anus sits a small area of connective tissue, the perineum. A lot of women like pressure here during penetration, and licking or nibbling during cunnilingus. This tissue is also somewhat elastic—it stretches during childbirth to allow passage of a baby's head. During her pregnancy, Susie Bright discovered that "perineal massage" recommended by her childbirth preparation teacher was much like fist fucking. "I could see why immediately," she writes in *Susie Bright's Sexual Reality*. "A hand going inside my pussy is a little like a baby's head trying to move outside into the world. How exciting! For the first time I felt a surge of confidence about my chances for a successful labor."[2]

Anus

The anus is a very sensitive area, ripe for erotic play. In Victorian porn, it's called the "little rosebud." Made of delicate tissue, rich in nerve endings and blood vessels, the anus is quite responsive to sexual arousal.

The anus is guarded by two muscles—the external sphincter, which consists of voluntary muscle (you can flex these muscles), and the internal sphincter, which consists of involuntary muscles (they seem to open and close according to their own will—like blinking—though with practice, you can learn to relax these, too).

The anus is short, just an inch or two long, leading into the rectum, which is about four to six inches long, and ending in the rectosigmoidal junction, the opening to the sigmoid colon. From there, the colon leads to the intestines. The rectum offers no equivalent of the cervix; there's no stopping point. Things really can get lost in there, so precautions are a must when inserting an object into your anus. Dildos and butt plugs must have a flanged base (bigger at the base than the top), and insertive toys, like anal beads, must be securely fastened to their strings.

The tissue of the anus engorges with arousal and is quite expansive; you can fit a finger, a dildo or penis, a butt plug, or even a whole hand inside your butt. The lining of the anus and rectum is very, very delicate, and will tear easily—another reason to be extremely careful in choosing insertive anal toys.

In biological males, the prostate gland, located on the front wall of the rectum a few inches from the anal opening, responds to stimulation similarly to the G-spot. You can insert a finger into the rectum and use that come-hither motion to find a partner's prostate. Male-to-female transsexuals, both preop and postop, can enjoy prostate stimulation.

PC Muscles

Finally, the pubococcygeus (PC) muscles are the set of muscles that run through your pelvic area in a figure eight. These are the muscles you exercise when you stop the flow of urine midstream—or grip your lover's finger! Developing these muscles will heighten your experience of orgasm; prevent incontinence when laughing or sneezing, or in old age; and generally help you become more aware of sensations in all areas of your genitals. Kegel exercises (named for the gynecologist who popularized them) involve squeezing your muscles as if you were shutting off the flow of urine. Inhale as you contract your PC muscles; hold the contraction for several seconds; and then exhale as you relax. Do this ten times. Then push out ten times. Repeat. Do this daily—on the bus, in traffic, and during Nike commercials.

Breasts

Many of us enjoy breast play—so much so that it gets its own chapter in this book! Unless you have health concerns or plan to breastfeed, you may not have sought out information on the anatomy of your breasts.

Our breasts are composed mostly of breast tissue and fat. Although the size of your breasts is genetically determined, your breast size will change as you gain or lose weight. One breast may be larger than the other. The size or shape of your breasts has no bearing on their responsiveness to sexual stimulation.

The aureola surrounds the nipple; it's darker than the rest of the breast. The aureola darkens and swells in response to sexual stimulation. The nipple becomes erect when stimulated; some women's nipples invert when aroused (Dr. Susan Love calls these "shy" nipples).[3]

Breast sensitivity varies from woman to woman, as well as at different points in a woman's menstrual cycle and over the course of her lifetime. PMS (premenstrual syndrome) and pregnancy can intensify breast sensitivity, and menopause can lessen breast sensitivity. Women who have cystic breasts may find breast play very uncomfortable.

Sexual Response

How do you know when you're turned on? Does your clit throb? Can you feel a pulsing at the mouth of your vagina or at the opening of your anus? Do you feel nervous or fluttery? Do you notice small contractions of the sphincter muscles? Do you feel yourself getting wet? Do your nipples get erect? Are you aware of your nipples brushing against the fabric of your clothing? Can you smell your own juices?

You may be familiar with the Masters and Johnson model of sexual response. In the 1960s, William Masters and Virginia Johnson identified four stages of sexual response: *arousal, plateau, orgasm,* and *resolution.*[4] Theirs became the standard model of describing what happens when we're sexual. Helen Singer Kaplan added a fifth stage, *desire,* to the model; she posited that before there is arousal, there's desire.[5] In the 1980s, Joann Loulan joined the chorus, adding a

Rachel Pepper's Tips on Sex During Pregnancy

ORGASMS. During pregnancy, you may notice a difference in your orgasms. Increased blood flow to all your sexual organs may mean that your orgasms are longer and more intense. Women who have previously been unable to climax may be able to do so now. Still others may find that sex is a bit uncomfortable now, as excitement builds quickly but orgasm stays just out of reach.

IS PENETRATION OK? Penetration with fingers is considered quite safe. Penetration with dildos is usually safe in low-risk pregnancies. As with all vaginal penetration during pregnancy, avoid vigorous, hard thrusting, and stop at the slightest bit of discomfort. Many women lay off penetration entirely toward the end of their pregnancy as the baby moves further down the pelvis.

IS IT OK IF MY LOVER LIES ON TOP OF ME? This should not be a problem in early pregnancy. In later months it may be too uncomfortable for the pregnant woman to bear the weight of her partner. As the pregnant woman grows, Anne Semans urges couples to be more creative about trying different positions. The pregnant partner may be more comfortable on top, or you can try making love side by side.

IS FISTING SAFE? Fisting is the practice of inserting a whole hand inside a woman's vagina. I would not recommend fisting during pregnancy. One doctor I asked about this said that the pressure on the greatly engorged blood vessels could be dangerous to the mother's health. If you are determined to be fisted during pregnancy, make sure you are with a partner whom you trust (and who knows your body!), go very slowly and carefully, avoid deep, hard thrusting, and stop at the slightest bit of discomfort.

WHAT ABOUT ANAL SEX? Anal sex is also safe as long as you proceed carefully, avoid hard thrusting, and stop at the slightest bit of discomfort. Start small: a finger, a small butt plug, a slender dildo. Tristan Taormino, in her book *The Ultimate Guide to Anal Sex for Women,* writes, "It is safe to have anal sex if you are pregnant, although some women find that they cannot get in a comfortable position for anal stimulation." Taormino suggests that pregnant women be extra careful about preventing any bacteria from traveling from the anal area to the vagina. This includes being very fastidious about keeping sex toys clean. It may be prudent here to point out that the same holds true when you use the toilet, since any vaginal infections that may result are more complicated to treat while you are pregnant.

IS IT OK TO USE LUBE? A water-based lube is fine for vaginal penetration. Remember: Never use oil-based lubricants in your vagina.

WHAT ABOUT BONDAGE, PIERCING, CUTTING, AND WHIPPING? Even the most sexually adventurous women curtail any practice that may be unsafe during pregnancy. If you cannot live without this type of sex play, always let your partners know you are pregnant, lay off the heavy stuff like whipping, and stop at the first sign of discomfort. Bondage is not a good idea, as it can constrict blood flow and cause cramping. Basically, you are playing at your own risk, and the risk of your unborn child. Be careful!

WHAT IF I GET AN INFECTION? If you notice any burning sensations, discomfort, or smells during pregnancy, it is always best to get them checked out right away. Many symptoms may just be part of the discomforts of pregnancy, but if you have an infection, you will probably need treatment. Of course, you should always make sure anyone treating you for this or any other medical problem is aware that you are pregnant.

WHAT IF I GET AN STD WHILE I AM PREGNANT? While STDs are never pleasant, acquiring one during pregnancy is even more awful, because most can do harm to the fetus. You may also not be able to treat the disease in the same manner while pregnant because of the toxic nature of the medications. It is therefore best to err on the side of caution while you are pregnant and engage in safer sex, particularly if you have a new partner. In the United States, you will be tested at least once or twice during your pregnancy for STDs, and it is a good idea to get these tests even where they are not required. Your doctor will discuss treatment options with you if you are found to have an STD.

WILL IT HURT THE BABY? Many pregnant women instinctively shy away from sexual activities that may harm the fetus. And, says Anne Semans, that's probably a good thing. "If you're worried about a particular sexual practice, don't do it," she says. "Now is the time to err on the side of safety. One good fuck isn't worth the price of a baby."

While it's true that the baby is protected within the uterus, there are a few sexual activities that you should definitely avoid. While cunnilingus is generally fine, blowing air into the vagina is a big no-no, as it can cause an air bubble in the bloodstream called an air embolism, which can be life-threatening to the mother. However, this is a rare condition and

not one that will come about as a result of regular sex play.

Anything that can damage the cervix is off-limits, including rough sex of any kind, thrusting too-large dildos inside you, and aggressive fisting.

On the other hand, my midwife Deborah Simone, of Awakenings Birth Services, says that a good, hearty session of sex may be just what a pregnant gal needs once in a while. She recommends staying away from deep thrusting into the vagina but says that making love doggie-style with penetration of the pregnant partner from behind may have its beneficial aspects. "It's a great way to get your perineum massage," says Simone of this position.

If you have concerns or questions regarding sex during pregnancy, it will probably be up to you to initiate a conversation with your health care provider. Very few physicians will be knowledgeable about the specifics of lesbian sex during pregnancy. For instance, if a doctor says "no sex" does that mean no penetration? No oral sex? No orgasm? Be prepared to ask explicit questions.

Instead of giving up on sex, empower yourself with some sex-positive information and support.

CAN SEX INDUCE LABOR? You may feel some contractions after sex, especially toward the very end of your pregnancy. This may make you anxious that labor could be triggered by lovemaking. While it's true that some midwives tell their clients to have sex or at least stimulate the nipples to bring on labor, this can really only happen if it's time for labor to begin anyway. However, if you are having a high-risk pregnancy, you may want to abstain from most sexual activity during the last few weeks.

sixth stage: *willingness*. Loulan, working with lesbian couples, offered the idea that even if there wasn't desire, there could be a willingness to feel desire.[6] Don't worry if your sexual response fails to follow any of the models. Human sexuality varies greatly from person to person, and even from day to day.

So why would it be useful to have a model of sexual response? Well, knowing generally how human sexual response works can help you understand your *own* experience. You can learn to notice your own sexual rhythms. Then you can decide what aspects of your sexual response you might like to develop more. Models such as these can give you a language to help you describe your experience, one that others may understand. However, if theories bore you—or, worse, make you feel inadequate—just skip them. You don't have to be a sexologist to have a fabulous sex life.

Understanding your own sexual response, however, *will* help you create a fabulous sex life. Try masturbating in front of a full-length mirror, or with a hand mirror between your legs. As you stimulate yourself, you'll get to see your particular sexual responses in action. You can become acquainted with the visual cues of your sexual arousal. (You can even insert a speculum—available from women's health centers and some sex-toy stores, such as Toys in Babeland (see "Resources")—and grab a flashlight to see what you look like on the inside when you're turned on.)

During arousal, your heart rate and blood pressure increase. You may feel warm. A sexual flush may appear over your face and chest. The breasts enlarge. Your nipples become erect; later in arousal, your aureola swell and your nipples may seem to retract. The clitoris engorges with blood and becomes erect, growing bigger. The inner labia swell and darken in color. You get wet. Your vaginal walls lubricate and the whole vagina expands. The uterus engorges and lifts, expanding up to twice its normal (not pregnant) size. Your vagina opens. Your sphincter muscles may relax or contract.

A friend once told me that women originally wore lipstick to symbolize the sexual engorgement of their lips during arousal—a reasonable explanation of why women who wore bright red lipstick were said to be "loose." Whether or not the story is true, my friend (happily) now can't look at a woman's freshly painted lips without thinking of the engorgement—and resulting darkening and deepening of color—during arousal.

The plateau stage is the state of peak excitement right before orgasm. The vagina opens up and balloons out. The clitoral glans is tucked inside its hood. The aureola continue to swell. You may notice that you can take more nipple stimulation. Muscle tension increases all throughout the body, as the heart rate continues to climb. You find yourself breathing faster and deeper. The sex flush becomes more pronounced. The labia minor may turn a deep red or wine color. The vagina opens into what's called the orgasmic platform. The outer one-third of the vagina further congests with blood.

Orgasm is a series of involuntary muscle contractions in the vagina, uterus, and anus, releasing the blood that's been stored in the erectile tissues of the genitals. Most sources report that the contractions occur at a rate of slightly more than one per second; generally an orgasm will involve anywhere from just a few contractions to 10 or 15 of them. Of course, the intensity and duration of the orgasm will vary greatly. During orgasm the heart rate peaks. Breathing is faster.

Resolution is the stage in which the body returns to its nonaroused state. You experience a release of tension. The heart rate and breathing return to normal. Sex flush disappears, nipple erection fades, the glans of the clit once again protrudes from its hood. The labia return to their nonaroused color and size.

Do women get "blue balls"—that painful state of unresolved arousal that men talk about? Yes—if after reaching a very high degree of arousal you don't come, it takes a longer time for the vascular congestion to ease, which can be uncomfortable—or exciting!

I love my cunt, for sure—the way its lips pucker, the way it hungers to get some. My cunt and I are partners in crime! Arrest us for being too hot!

Orgasm

Orgasm is leaving my body and coming back anew.

So, *orgasms!* You can have orgasm-directed sex by yourself or with a partner. If it's all about getting off, that's fine. You can also have sex without orgasm, and that's fine, too. Most of us want that release of coming. We yearn to "give it up."

Many women are completely happy with our orgasmic capacity. Others want to come harder, quicker, longer, more easily, more often, more transcendently, or more meaningfully. You may wonder if you're doing it "right"—and you may have had lovers who pressured you to respond differently than was natural for you.

You *can* enhance your capacity for orgasm—and you'll find plenty of tips and techniques throughout this book to help you do just that. In fact, here's the first one: *You're fine just the way you are.* Even if you've never had an orgasm, you're not defective in any way. Your experience of sexual pleasure is uniquely yours and no less valid than anyone else's. Sex is not a competitive sport.

I would love to be able to have an orgasm more easily than I do. But when I have them they are incredibly intense.

Do you start coming as the first drop of moisture hits your panties? Perhaps you come ten seconds after the vibrator touches your clit, and you don't feel complete until you've come nonstop for an hour. Good for you!

I orgasm and cum very easily. Just the brush of a woman's wet tongue on my clitoris causes me to orgasm.

I can come every few minutes for several hours.

Do the words "Pillow Princess" ring a bell? Or "Do-Me Queen"? So what if you don't consider one or two (or three or four or five!) orgasms sufficient? Even if every dyke you've ever loved has had to seek medical intervention for repetitive stress injury, there's nothing wrong with you. How much pleasure is too much? It's *your* call.

This Is Taking Too Long

Perhaps your partners have complained that you're a "hard come," taking too long to reach orgasm. Too long for whom? If it takes 30 minutes of perfect clit stimulation, with just the right touch in just the right spot, for you to reach orgasm, you're fine. Enjoy the attention.

If you'd like to come more quickly or reliably, however, here are six specific techniques you might try:

- Experiment with different positions or activities. Switch from oral sex to penetration or clitoral stimulation. Get on top. Find out what works for you.
- Make sure you're really turned on before you even *think* of attempting to come. Human sexual response isn't linear. Back off, do something else, and then come back to your arousal.
- Buy a vibrator. Many women find the strong, consistent stimulation of a vibrator to be the most sure-fire aid to achieving orgasm.
- Touch yourself. Play with your clit while your girl's going down on you, while she's penetrating you, even while she's touching you.
- Breathe into your pelvis, move your pelvis, don't clench—let go.
- Fantasize. What are the images or scenarios that make you sizzle? It's OK to fantasize during partner sex.

If you come only by your own hand or vibrator, you're no less a sexual partner. You can incorporate masturbation into partner sex in a way that will be incredibly hot for both you and your partner. You'll find suggestions throughout the book for what to do when your lover's tongue or hands—or even her strap-on—get tired. (These will also help out with your partner's fatigue and that pesky repetitive stress problem.)

> I need my vibrator; it's very difficult for me to come by any other method. I can have an orgasm from oral sex, but it's hard for my girlfriend to keep up the constant, unchanging stimulation that I need. I need repetitive movements, and it takes a while.

If you don't happen to have an earth-shattering orgasm every time your girlfriend makes love to you, it doesn't mean that she's a bad lover or that you've fallen out of love. It may be that you're just not getting the right stimulation to send you over the edge. You might be too stressed. You may not know your partner well enough, trust her enough, trust *yourself* enough, or feel safe enough to give it up in that moment. Just how vulnerable you care to be varies from day to day.

> *I don't always have the most intense orgasms that I know I can have. It depends on my psychological readiness to be thoroughly opened.*

Orgasm is about pleasure. It's not about your girlfriend's reputation or bedpost notches (that's *her* problem). That she may be gratified by your coming is great—but it's not the point for you.

However you come, how easily, how hard, how often, you have a sexuality that's yours and yours alone. You're not broken, gluttonous, selfish, oversexed, defective, or perverted (unless thinking of yourself in these terms turns you on!). You needn't compare yourself to some mythic example of Sapphic perfection.

How Do You Come?

How do you reach orgasm? Women come from all sorts of stimulation. Most women require clitoral stimulation to reach orgasm—from vibrators, fingers, tongues, or surfaces to rub up against.

Many women find nothing sends them into orbit quite like a tongue and lips licking, sucking, and nibbling on their clit. For others, oral sex is just not intense enough to bring them to orgasm.

> *The tried-and-true tongue-to-clit method is still the only thing besides my Hitachi Magic Wand that never fails to bring me to orgasm.*

Many women come from penetration—either vaginal or anal—without any clitoral stimulation at all.

> *The first time I came with a partner, it was a vaginal orgasm—my girlfriend was finger fucking me. That's still how I come best, and I can have many, many orgasms in a row that way.*

Others find their orgasms are intensified when clitoral stimulation is combined with penetration, either vaginal or anal.

I don't come without clitoral stimulation. But when vaginal penetration is added, it's like a deeper experience; it reaches into my insides and clenches with intense pleasure.

Different kinds of stimulation produce difference experiences of orgasm. Some women make clear distinctions between the orgasms they experience from clitoral stimulation versus penetration.

Vaginal orgasms feel as if they happen deeper in my body; they feel more like contractions. A clitoral orgasm is sharper, more like an intense tingling that spreads over my body. I'm multiorgasmic, and I need one of each to feel really satisfied.

Some women reach orgasm with sufficient attention to their nipples. Others come from fantasy and mental stimulation. Tantra practitioners move erotic energy through their bodies, experiencing energy or body orgasms.

I have very intense concentration and my mind becomes my orgasm. I can ride it for a fairly long time.

Some women come from pain and other intense sensations of S/M play—and some tops are known to come simply from administering to their bottoms.

My favorite way to come is from caning someone. We don't need any other contact but the cane with her ass, to make me come—if I can hurt her enough. I come from doing, rather than from being done.

I can come from pain. From clitoral stimulation. From hard fucking or fisting. I can come just from having my nipples pinched hard. I can come from sufficient mental stimulation with no body contact.

Getting Her Off

I love orchestrating someone else's orgasm.

Rarely do sex guides give sufficient attention to the pleasures of facilitating another's orgasm. Discussions of orgasm are typically about *getting* them, not *giving* them. Yet getting a partner off is central to lesbian sex. It's thrilling to feel a woman come in your mouth, to find yourself gripped between her powerful thighs, or to feel her vaginal contractions clamp down on your hand.

Taking turns pleasuring one another is a wonderful way to enjoy sex. But not all women have reciprocity as their goal. What if your partner doesn't want to have an orgasm? Does that mean she identifies as a "stone butch"? Maybe. Maybe not. Why not ask her? You can't predict gender identity by whether or not someone is orgasm-focused. See Chapter 12, "Gender and (Not Destiny)." It also doesn't necessarily mean she's shut down, self-hating, or unable to have orgasms.

Ask your partner how she feels about orgasm and what kinds of sexual attention she likes for herself. She may share with you profound feelings about her gender and sexuality. She may feel completely gratified by your sexual encounter. After your strap-on stud has finished riding you through more orgasms than you can count, she may simply be spent.

> *Truly, all I care about is pleasing my femme. Sometimes I don't have any orgasms at all, and neither one of us feels that the session is missing anything. Now, if my girlfriend didn't have an orgasm, I imagine that we would feel differently—but that's only because she really, really wants me to get her off. We have different sexual roles.*

Your partner's experience of your orgasm isn't vicarious. Think of your partner's lips, hand, or pelvis as a conduit for sexual energy. As your body is humming with orgasm, your partner is riding that wave with you. She may indeed feel your orgasm from her heart to the bottom of her toes.

Multiple Orgasms

Women can and do have multiple orgasms. Which doesn't mean you *should* have multiple orgasms or even that multiple orgasms are more satisfying than ordinary single orgasms.

> *I'm not multiorgasmic and that's OK with me because the ones I already have nearly break the bank.*

But many women do find that one orgasm leads to another, with very little time elapsing in between.

> *After being fucked really hard, if my partner goes back to my clitoris and plays roughly with it, I will usually orgasm again, and again, and again....*

Rather than relaxing into afterglow, these women go right back to the plateau stage and come over and over. Some women experience this as a series of smaller orgasms; others experience orgasms that increase in intensity and duration, leading up to a really big bang.

> *Sometimes I have smaller orgasms before the big one. After the big one, I get ticklish and it's hard to be touched. But if my partner works past that point I have powerful orgasms over and over.*

How do you achieve multiple orgasms? In *The New Good Vibrations Guide to Sex*, Cathy Winks and Anne Semans offer three rules for achieving multiple orgasms: "back off, breathe, and move." After you come, and your clit is too sensitive to touch, back off without entirely ceasing stimulation. Winks and Semans suggest switching to a lighter or less-direct touch. Then, breathe. Breathing oxygenates your body and keeps the energy flowing. And move—move your pelvis, your legs, your feet. "Let the energy build back up in your genitals. Within a few minutes, excruciating overstimulation may well give way to excruciating pleasure...." [7]

> *The only way I reach multiple orgasms is if my partner just doesn't stop when I tell her to. Then they're in rapid-fire succession.*

Extended Orgasms

You may experience extended orgasms, one long delicious coming that seems to last and last. Or you may ride the edge of the plateau almost indefinitely, without actually coming.

What if orgasm wasn't a peak (sharp rise, sharp drop) but a wave or flow of sensation and energy? Margo Anand, author of the classic *The Art of Sexual Ecstasy: The Path of Sacred Sexuality for Western Lovers*, suggests that instead of thinking of orgasm as an *explosion*—sending energy outward—we think of it as an *implosion* and redirect the energy upward and through the chakras, or energy centers, of the body.[8]

Mikaya Heart distinguishes between multiple and extended orgasms. In her book *When the Earth Moves: Women and Orgasm*, she defines extended orgasm as a state of "continual sensation" that can last up to six hours, while multiple orgasms are discrete "ongoing individual orgasms with a break between each one, and then more stimulation to bring on the next one."[9]

If you prefer the "big bang" to the continual wave, you might actually find extended orgasm frustrating. But if you want to experience a long, unfolding ride, you may want to learn more about Tantric practices.

Ejaculation

> *I like to ejaculate. I mean, I can really flood the bed.*

Female ejaculate is produced in the paraurethral glands. Ejaculate isn't urine, though it may contain small traces of urine. The clear fluid may contain vaginal lubrication, cervical mucus, and fluid from the uterus, and may have a similar chemical composition to male ejaculate (minus the sperm).

How much fluid is ejaculated varies from woman to woman. Some women spurt streams of ejaculate into the air. Others leave a pie-sized puddle on the sheets. The amount of lubrication we produce is quite individual and is affected by menstrual cycle, age, health conditions, and even medications like antihistamines.

A lot of women feel self-conscious about what they perceive to be peeing during sex, mistaking ejaculate for urine. You can reassure yourself by urinating before sex.

For some women, ejaculation precedes orgasm. They experience a gush of wetness right before orgasm. For others, ejaculation and orgasm are separate phenomena. Ejaculation may be experienced as a feeling of release with a nice big spray of come—but not the same level of intensity as other orgasms. This may or may not feel satisfying.

Some women like having sex with women who gush or ejaculate; others find it a big mess. Place a waterproof pad (you'll find them in the incontinence aisle of your local pharmacy) under a towel to protect your bed.

Much has been written lately about "G-spot orgasms"—orgasms resulting from G-spot stimulation and accompanied by ejaculation. Some women ejaculate with G-spot stimulation. Some ejaculate without any penetration at all. Others simply don't ejaculate.

How can you learn to ejaculate? You can explore your urethral sponge or G-spot with a firm curved dildo or your fingers (particularly if you have long arms or a short torso or are particularly flexible!). Make sure you're well-aroused. (One review of the scientific literature regarding female ejaculation, published in the *Archives of Sexual Behavior*, cited "full tumescence" of the vagina as a requirement for ejaculation.[10]) Insert your fingers or dildo, aiming for the front (anterior) wall of the vagina. Stroke this area with a "come hither" motion. If you use your fingers, you'll feel the difference in texture between this area, which is rough, and the rest of the vaginal walls, which are smooth. Some women like to stimulate the opening of the vagina just below the urethra. You can also press down on your pelvis with your free hand, applying pressure just above the pubic bone. Stimulate your G-spot until you feel intensely turned on and like you're about to pee. As you approach orgasm, push out, as if urinating. The stream you produce is ejaculate.

If you'd like to learn more about the G-spot and ejaculation, read *The Good Vibrations Guide to the G-Spot* by Cathy Winks. This brief guide packs solid information on female sexual anatomy and sexual techniques. You might also want to investigate how-to videos—such Fanny Fatale's *How to Female Ejaculate*. The Web links at the end of this chapter will lead you to sources of recent research on female ejaculation.

Please *include something on the topic of female ejaculation. I had a horrible experience last year in a damn Ivy League graduate school (social work) class with a professor who, in a course on human behavior in the social environment, made a big deal about how teenage boys masturbate more and are more sexually aware than girls* because they have visible results. *I contacted her outside the class to cite some textual evidence on female ejaculation (rather than anecdotal evidence), and she basically dismissed it all with the valid point that there simply hasn't been enough research published on the matter....*

Why am I interested in this? Well, my lover is a kick-ass ejaculator. Not all the time, but on demand. If I ask her to squirt for me, it usually happens. It's quick, and quiet, and quite arousing. Just at the point of orgasm, she gets very wet, but not normal wet...more like water, and my hand gets kinda prune-ish, like when I've been in the bath too long, and then it's a sudden O, after which there's a big ole wet spot on the sheets. Love it. How she knew she could is beyond me...We were talking once and she said very casually that she thought she could ejaculate, but that she'd been afraid of it, and always managed to hold back during orgasm. The next time we made love, I asked her if she would let it all out for me, and she did. Amazing.

If You Can't Have an Orgasm

If you've never had an orgasm, or aren't sure if you've had an orgasm, you may be preorgasmic, a term that presumes that you *can* become orgasmic. (See Chapter 5, "Masturbation," for suggestions on learning to orgasm.) There are many reasons why you may never have had an orgasm or may find it very difficult to reach orgasm. Chief among them are lack of information about your body and sexual response, dissociation, and trauma from sexual abuse. You may be *anorgasmic* (not having orgasms) for physiological reasons. These include a range of health conditions—and the medications used to treat them.

Illness and Disability

Any disability, medical condition, or medical treatment that affects blood pressure, blood flow, muscles, or nerves can affect one's ability to orgasm. These may include diabetes, muscular sclerosis, spinal injuries, and high blood pressure. Nerve damage can affect the sensitivity of the clitoris, making it either numb or too painful to touch. Some women suffer from over-sensitivity. For seemingly no reason, their clit or nipples are too sensitive to be touched at all. Conditions like Attention Deficit Disorder (ADD) that interfere with one's ability to concentrate can make orgasm difficult.

Hidden disabilities can have a particularly frustrating impact on sexuality. Feeling fine one day, but having genital touching be painful the next, can make it very difficult to sustain interest in a sex life.

Surviving cancer and the treatments for it can affect sexuality. Many women who undergo chemotherapy experience a chemically induced premature menopause, with all the associated symptoms, like loss of vaginal lubrication and elasticity.

Aging

Yes, the older I get the harder it is for me to have orgasms. I also don't think they are as strong or satisfying as they used to be.

The New Ourselves Growing Older reports a number of age-related changes in sexual response and sexual anatomy. These include reduction in vaginal lubrication, slower arousal time, less-intense vaginal and uterine contractions, and changes in the vagina: "As we age the lips of the vagina, or the labia, become less firm…the length of the vagina may seem shorter, since the tissues are less elastic." [12] Penetration may become painful or irritating as the thinning vaginal tissues provide less cushioning for the urethra and bladder. Now's the time to experiment with lube (if you haven't already) and to explore new ways of enjoying sexuality.

Lubrication

Often the first sign of arousal many of us notice is lubrication. So, if we don't lubricate, we may not "feel" aroused. Lubrication, of course, is affected by our menstrual cycle, aging (with the loss of estrogen in menopause, many women lubricate less), and medications—even antihistamines can dry you up.

Sex and Depression

Nothing kills an otherwise healthy sex life like depression.

Depression can severely diminish libido. It's hard to muster much interest in sex when you're barely getting through the day. Even more frustrating for many women is that some medications available to treat depression can often affect sexual desire and functioning. Some women report that antidepressants cause a dip in desire; others report an inability to orgasm or a muted quality to their orgasms. Not all women experience sexual side effects while on antidepressants. Some notice no change whatsoever. For many women, just not being depressed kick-starts their libido enough to overcome the effects of antidepressants. But for those who do experience side effects, they're a real problem. It's disheartening to finally come alive again—only to feel robbed of one's capacity for erotic pleasure.

Antidepressants or Orgasm Suppressants?

Most notorious for negative sexual side affects are the SSRIs (selective serotonin reuptake inhibitors), the class of drugs most frequently prescribed for depression. While medications like Paxil, Prozac, Zoloft, and others have helped many overcome debilitating depression (and no doubt saved many lives), they have also been known to cause sexual problems in some who take them.

Psychiatrists and other physicians have come up with a few tricks, such as combining two different antidepressants—for instance, coupling an SSRI with another type of antidepressant, such as Wellbutrin, that doesn't seem to adversely affect sexual functioning. They can also closely monitor patients to find the precise dosage that ameliorates the symptoms of depression while minimizing adverse side effects. Landing on a treatment that works for you can take months of persistent effort—no small task for someone suffering from depression.

Health care practitioners have come up with other creative solutions as well. Some recommend testosterone patches for women, used in conjunction with an SSRI. Small doses of testosterone administered through the skin can add a bit of zip to the libido, they say—without leading to increased body hair or other secondary male sex characteristics. Likewise, some women who take SSRIs report an increase in libido when combined with Dehydroepiandrosterone (DHEA), an adrenal hormone used by bodybuilders. (DHEA use has also been linked to acne and mood swings as well.) There hasn't been adequate research on DHEA or testosterone to know whether long-term use by women will lead to health problems.

Researchers are studying the potential of Viagra to help women who report negative sexual side effects from SSRIs ("iatrogenic serotonergic antidepressant medication-induced sexual dysfunction,"[11] to those in the know). They're studying the possibilities for postmenopausal women as well. While Viagra (sildenafil) was developed to help men overcome erectile dysfunction, it's increasingly being taken by women who experience difficulty reaching orgasm. Viagra is a relatively short-acting medication. You can take Viagra before the Big Date, but it won't restore the ongoing flow of erotic energy in your life.

Some women who suffer from depression have found it helpful to combine lower dosages of an SSRI with St. John's wort or other herbal and nutritional remedies such as yohimbe and gingko. Others have abandoned SSRIs altogether, favoring these alternative strategies.

Of course, decisions regarding management of depression should be made with the help of a health care practitioner who is knowledgeable about the available treatments and respectful of the needs of lesbian, bisexual, and transsexual patients. For many of us, that is easier said than done.

Finding Help

Most physicians spend less time learning about human sexuality—roughly 12 hours of classroom instruction—than you spent learning to drive a car. Homophobia may creep into the doctor/patient relationship in a variety of ways. Your physician may downplay your concerns about your sex life. She or he may feel uncomfortable talking to you about sex between women (or any sex at all). Your physician may view lesbians as not sexually "active"—since they presume we're not having sex with men. More subtly, it might be assumed that if you're not partnered, you aren't interested in having sex.

Of course, many health care practitioners do quite well with lesbian, bisexual, and transsexual patients—especially since so many of us fill the ranks of the health care industry. Now that sexual side effects of antidepressants have gained such notoriety, many health care practitioners have become quite comfortable discussing libido and medication. Whether

you're seeking the help of a psychiatrist, physician, or therapist, the best strategy for reclaiming your libido is to find someone who will work with you. Here are some questions to ask yourself when choosing a health care professional:

- Do you get a gut sense that this practitioner will treat you respectfully— regardless of your gender identity or sexual choices?

- Do you feel comfortable talking to this practitioner? Does she or he listen to you?

- Does this practitioner have other lesbian, bisexual, or transsexual patients or clients? Who's recommending this individual?

- Is the practitioner qualified to answer your questions regarding the best course of treatment for your depression?

- How many hours of formal training in human sexuality has this practitioner received?

- Does the practitioner support you in prioritizing sexual satisfaction in your sex life?

Resources such as Kink Aware Professionals (www.bannon.com/kap) provide referrals to health care professionals who are sensitive to the needs of lesbians, gays, transsexuals, sex workers, and S/M and fetish devotees. The "Resources" section of this book lists many helpful contacts for those seeking support and care. Your local women's or queer community center may also provide referrals to health care professionals.

If you aren't lubricating, you may think you're not turned on. What to do? Well, for starters, invest in your sexual pleasure by purchasing some lube! (More on lube in Chapter 15, "Sex Toys and Accoutrements.")

Second, start noticing your other signs of arousal. Do your nipples harden and become more sensitive? Do you feel a fluttering in your belly? Can you feel your PC muscles contract?

Finally, ask yourself how *you* feel about your capacity for pleasure. Want to come faster? Want to take longer? Want to have deeper, more satisfying orgasms? Want to come more than once in a night? For more than 30 seconds? What's important is that *you* develop your sexuality in directions that bring you the most pleasure—regardless of what others may think or what you've been told is possible for you.

Suggested Web Links:

THE CLITORIS.COM
    www.the-clitoris.com
FEMALE EJACULATION AND THE G-SPOT
    www8.tripnet.se/~eidos/female_ejaculation/articles.html
FEMALE EJACULATION BIBLIOGRAPHY
    www.incontinet.com/ejacbib.htm

NOTES
1. Susan Williamson, reporting O'Connell's findings in *Today's Life Science*. See also Helen E. O'Connell, et al., "Anatomical Relationship Between Urethra and Clitoris," *Journal of Urology*, vol. 159, 1892–97, June 1999.
2. Susie Bright, *Susie Bright's Sexual Reality* (Cleis Press, 1992), 102.
3. Dr. Susan Love with Karen Lindsey, *Dr. Susan Love's Breast Book*, 2d ed. (Perseus Books, 1995), 5.
4. William Masters and Virginia Johnson, *Human Sexual Response* (Lippincott Williams & Wilkins, 1966).
5. Helen Singer Kaplan, *The New Sex Therapy* (out of print, 1974).
6. Joann Loulan, *Lesbian Sex* (Spinsters, 1984) and *Lesbian Passion* (Spinsters, 1987).
7. Cathy Winks and Anne Semans, *The New Good Vibrations Guide to Sex* (Cleis Press, 1997), 28.
8. Margo Anand, *The Art of Sexual Ecstasy: The Path of Sacred Sexuality for Western Lovers* (Tarcher, 1989), 309.
9. Mikaya Heart, *When the Earth Moves: Women and Orgasm* (Celestial Arts, 1998), 109.
10. Carol Ann Darling, J. Kenneth Davidson, Sr., and Colleen Conway-Welch, "Female Ejaculation: Perceived Origins, the Grafenberg Spot/Area, and Sexual Responsiveness," *Archives of Sexual Behavior*, vol. 19, no. 1, 45, 1990.
11. H. G. Nurnberg, et al., "Sildenafil for iatrogenic serotonergic antidepressant medication-induced sexual dysfunction in 4 patients," *Journal of Clinical Psychiatry*, vol. 60, no. 1, 33–35, January 1999.
12. Paula B. Doress-Worters and Diana Laskin Siegal, *The New Ourselves Growing Older* (Touchstone, 1994), 89.

SOURCE OF SIDEBAR
Rachel Pepper, *The Ultimate Guide to Pregnancy for Lesbians* by Rachel Pepper (Cleis Press, 1999).

chapter four

The Road to Heaven Leads to You

I love my body! At least, I try to.
It's my goal to say I love my body and really mean it.

HOW DO YOU FEEL ABOUT YOUR BODY? Many of us love our bodies. We love our strength and passion, and we love the pleasure we take in our flesh. We love our broad backs and strong thighs, love the way our bodies carry us through life. We love our full, rich lips, sharp teeth, and piercing eyes. We love our boyish smiles and lean bodies, love our well-defined muscles that ripple as we move. We love the dark berries of our nipples, the ripe plum swelling of our cunts. We love our graceful hands, the delicate slope from neck to shoulder and from waist to hip. We love our voluptuously long legs. We love our eagerness, our openness, the desire that gushes from our vulvas. We love our roundness: round face, round breasts, round belly, round butt, round thighs, the generosity of flesh we offer up to our lovers.

I honestly like my body. Please publish that in your book. Some of us just really like our bodies.

It's marvelous how much delight we take in our bodies. When you consider the ridiculously narrow cultural standards most people hold for female beauty, it's truly remarkable that so many of us wholeheartedly love our bodies. Do you ever get the feeling that if you give yourself a compliment, someone will correct you? ("Dream on, girlfriend—those cellulite bags are *not* becoming!") You might even think it impolite or conceited to say you find yourself gorgeous. It may seem safer to downplay the whole thing.

> *My body is beautiful. I have never had to worry about weight, and I am athletic, so therefore muscular. If anything, my love of my body is not the norm, so consequently I conceal this love most of the time and feign shyness when complimented. I think of my body as one of the bonus prizes a lover of mine gets…a beautifully sculpted woman's body to play with.*

No matter what your size, shape, age, health concerns, abilities or disabilities, HIV or STD status, you deserve to love yourself fully and unconditionally—and that includes your body.

A Love/Hate Relationship

So many of us women come to adulthood with less than perfect feelings about our bodies. Even if our families were supportive of how we looked and felt, our commodity-oriented, gender-obsessed, homophobic, *and* lesbophobic culture probably was not!

Many of us continue to feed a love/hate relationship with our bodies. We accept and reject parts of ourselves, managing only a cafeteria-style kind of acceptance.

> *Some days I can't keep the internalized stuff in check. I hate it…my body. Belly's fat. Butt ain't big and bubbly enuff for a Black girl. More breasts. Less breasts. Skin too dark. Skin too light. On these days I just can't win! I don't have many days like this—thank Gawd!*

Finding out that others love exactly the characteristics of your body you'd like to hide can be quite an awakening. That belly? That butt? You may have gotten the message that it all adds up to something less than zero—but odds are some women are out there who'd be tickled to look just like you (and to take you to bed!).

Many of us come to love ourselves in spite of severe barriers—such as childhood sexual abuse, eating disorders, addiction, depression, disability, chronic or life-threatening illnesses, or harassment for our gender presentation or sexual choices. Add racism and classism, and the mix gets very thick. For us, developing a positive self-image is a lifelong process, with a fully conscious relationship with our bodies as our reward. Our self-love is hard won and thus all the more precious.

Formerly ignored, stuffed, and numbed with food, I love my body. What aspects of my body make me happy? That everything I have pretty much keeps me alive and kicking to enjoy another day.

Body size, of course, is the most common stumbling block women mention when they talk about body image. Too fat. Too thin. We've been trained to measure our self-worth according to the numbers on the scale.

My mother used to tell me that no one would ever find me beautiful unless I lost weight, and it wasn't until I met the love of my life that I finally stopped believing it.

Skinny femme girl that I am, there are times I've wished for a more womanly figure. But I love that my small breasts disappear in the palms of my lover's hands—and the ease with which I am lifted into her arms. I love catching butch girls staring at my braless chest, my nipples peeking out though a thin shirt.

I like my broad shoulders, big hands, tight ass. I enjoy being strong. I love being able to pick up my lover, wrap her around my waist, and fuck her even longer than she thought she wanted.

Weight issues get complicated by gender and sexual orientation. It's disconcerting to be told that because you are delicate and petite, you can't possibly be a dyke (after all, *you* could get a man)—or that because you're big and broad-shouldered, you could *only* be a dyke (because no man would have you). Thankfully, many of us manage to turn this around.

I am big-boned, with quarterback shoulders, muscular biceps, and calves an NFL pro kicker would die for.

I'm a fat dyke. That used to be an issue for me but it isn't any more. My hills and valleys and breasts make an excellent playground for those who are adventurous enough to explore them.

During the process of gender transition, body image takes on a whole new layer of meaning. What does it mean to identify as masculine when you have 40DD breasts? To be female but not feminine? To wear your clit as a cock? Or conversely, to be 45 years old and have the brand-new budding breasts of a 14-year-old girl? To identify as female and have a penis?

For years, sex was unsatisfying for me because I was completely out of touch with my body. Now that I'm in the early stages of transitioning from female to male, I can handle physical pleasure and accept that this flesh-cart is part of me.

My breasts are small but perky, and I love my tattoos and my nipple piercing. I have a beautiful tattoo of ivy on my breast covering scars from a lumpectomy I had when I was 19. It made me feel so much better about my breasts when I had that done!

Take a Good Look

Get naked and position yourself in front of a full-length mirror. Lights up! Take an uncritical look at yourself. Drop your judgments, save your critical skills for a film review, and forget all the things you've heard about what you are "supposed" to look like. Just look at yourself. Pay attention. What do you see?

I have a nice hourglass shape (maybe a two-hour glass!) and my breasts are full, which I like. I like how I look without clothes because I pretty much like how anyone looks without clothes—we're all so unique and interesting and vulnerable and human without clothes.

Appreciate Yourself

I love that I'm so sensitive! Everything feels so damn good!

Masturbation is a great way to appreciate yourself. If you want to challenge yourself, masturbate in front of the mirror. You can stand, sit in a chair or on the floor, or lie on your side. Try to maintain eye contact with your image in the mirror—at least until you get too turned on to focus at all! More on masturbation tips and techniques in Chapter 5, "Masturbation."

Take It In

Next time someone pays you a compliment, take it in. All the way in. Don't toss it off, don't disagree, don't make excuses. Say, "Thank you." Period. Let yourself be appreciated. Of course, no one can talk you into believing you are beautiful—and you'll get nowhere if your self-esteem hinges on others' approval. Yet it's nice to know somebody likes how you look. Being showered with compliments never hurts!

I feel a lot better about my body than I used to. Part of it is that I got in shape, part of it is my lover's appreciation of my body. She plays it like a goddamn violin.

Join the Crowd

How often do you have the opportunity to appreciate other women's bodies? Next time you are in an environment where women are naked—whether it's the locker room or your favorite swimming hole—take a good look. Appreciate the variety of shapes and sizes. No judgments, no evaluations, and no comparing!

One reason we're so critical of ourselves is that we are isolated. We don't get to see enough naked bodies to view ourselves as unique (but really not-so-unique) members of humanity. That's one of the amazing contributions of the women's music festivals—being naked with thousands of naked women who span every possible description, and some that you've never even thought of.

The locker room is reason enough for a trip to the gym. If you hit the right gym at the right time of day (try a downtown YWCA at lunchtime), you'll find a diverse group of women whose bodies take all shapes.

When I'm feeling less than wonderful about my body, I take a trip to my local women's bathhouse, which offers a hot tub, sauna, steam room, outdoor deck, and massage. (It's not a women's bathhouse in the sexual sense of the term, though I'm sure that would be very popular in my town.)

You might think it counterintuitive to be naked in public on a bad body-image day—"What? You want me to show off *this* body?!"—but it really helps. The first 20 minutes are excruciating—and not because of the temperature of the hot tub! After a while, all those judgments peel away like so much dead skin. Your bones get the message, even if your head is skeptical. You may surprise yourself and feel infinitely better by the time you leave. Many cities have women's baths or public baths with women-only days.

Finally, my favorite place to stare at naked bodies is actually the one place where such behavior is socially appropriate—and even encouraged. Sex parties and sex clubs provide great lessons in humanity. All those naked people! Such

My body is femme, fat, cushy, strong, pale, soft—I love it. It's just right.

abundant flesh! The smells of women's arousal mingling with sweat. The sounds of bodies slapping together, women laughing and coming. (And at S/M play parties, the sounds of floggers thudding against backs, paddles smacking buttocks, and big, hearty screams.) At a sex party, you'll see women you find less attractive than yourself being treated like sex goddesses. And you'll see women you find too stunning to approach getting no more (or less) attention than you. The "Resources," lists local contact information for group sex events.

Get Into Your Body

> *The more active I am, the more positive feelings I have for my body. It's nice to feel powerful—to feel how my body can move me around and give me joy, through lovers, self-love, running, kung-fu punching, and dancing.*

Move your body. Breathe. Feel your heart pumping. Let your skin heat up. Get into your body. Can you feel your bones? Muscles and tissue? You can learn how to feel yourself from the inside. You can do this whether you're athletic or not. Even if the closest you've ever come to meditation is a 20-minute nap, you can become conscious of yourself as a sensate being. You don't have to be able to get up out of your chair to have a positive relationship with your body.

Perhaps the most obvious (and readily available) form of body work is massage. Following a masseuse's hands as she works your body can help you become aware of every bit of you—from the backs of your knees to the wings of your shoulder blades. If you don't feel comfortable being touched by a stranger or can't afford a professional massage, you can trade with a good friend. This has the added advantage of giving you an opportunity to explore another person's body while enhancing your friendship.

Former shy girl Carol Queen recommends solo dancing. Get out of your clothes, pop in your favorite CD, and *move*. In *Exhibitionism for the Shy*, Queen writes, "Feel your body move; disconnect your head from all the worries about how you look, and concentrate on letting the music sink into your limbs…. Dancing can lead you into your body perhaps further than you've ever been before."[1]

Been dancing alone for too long? Hit the clubs! Go dancing. Not only will you get to move your body and shake that booty—you'll get out of the house. If you don't like to move to a club beat, find a swing, two-step, or country-and-western group.

Go to the gym. Not to "improve" your body—though you may enjoy water aerobics or power lifting—but to experience yourself inhabiting your body and to see other people doing it, too. You can take classes in yoga or kick-boxing—it doesn't matter, as long as you find an activity that works for you.

Don't like the gym? Go to the park. Walk. Get a skateboard. Ride your bike. Roll your chair along a different path. Take a new route to work, and walk there. The point is to engage in activity that will bring you into a relationship with your physical self. Sure, you'll find buff specimens in the park, but you'll also see people who look just like you.

If the parks and gyms in your town are too straight for comfort, start an all-dyke workout group. You can meet once or twice a week for long, brisk walks; hit the gym on the buddy system; sign up for a martial arts class (ask for a group discount!); or go swimming on your lunch hour.

Your body need not be a box you are locked into all by yourself.

Somatic Healing

> *I've had a long, hard struggle overcoming an abusive relationship that included sexual assault. Because of this, I haven't learned a lot about my sexuality that many people learn when they are younger, so I've had the nice experience of being an actual grown-up when I figured out what I was doing. Of course there have been negative consequences: I sometimes still have flashbacks during sex, even with my long-term partner.*

Somatic healers teach the concept that the body and mind are part of one intelligent biological system. Your emotions do not exist separate from your body. So if you "feel" less than gorgeous, the solution may lie in deepening your relationship with your body rather than trying to escape it.

Do you "check out" during sex? Do you think you'd have an easier time reaching orgasm if you could stop your mind from wandering? Or are you fine for a good fuck—as long as your partner doesn't get too emotionally close?

Emotions are part of your cellular history, your body's "memory" of where it has been. The feelings associated with a traumatic experience don't go away, even if we ignore them. Trauma remains in the body until the emotions surrounding it are resolved and integrated into your experience. Your body will continue to respond automatically to situations you perceive—from your body's perspective—to be threatening. One survival strategy is simply to shut down.

I have large breasts and they have little feeling. Little feeling in breast and vagina.... Thank goddess my clitoris is in working order. Otherwise I'd be a Barbie.

Regardless of what has caused your body to respond like a town under siege, the trauma remains. Whether you have survived childhood sexual abuse, emotional neglect, physical abuse, a battering adult relationship, rape, sexual harassment, queer bashing, a life-threatening accident or illness, or even time spent in a war zone, healing trauma is a slow, painful process. And it's the only way to get your *self* back.

Staci Haines, author of *The Survivor's Guide to Sex: How to Have an Empowered Sex Life After Child Sexual Abuse*, stresses somatic healing as the key to sexual healing:

Your body was a dangerous place.... Leaving your body then, or dissociating, was an intelligent move. The memories or experiences of the trauma are often still present or "held" in your body today. Many survivors stay out of their bodies and senses long after the danger has passed to avoid revisiting those stored experiences.

Yet, your body is also you. It is the place in which you live and are alive. You connect and are in relationship with others from your body. You act in the world from your body. Your body is where the healing from trauma and abuse happens. Your body is also where you experience sensual and sexual pleasure. To experience all of these pleasures, however, you must be in your body, or "embodied." [2]

Happily, you have many kinds of healing practices to choose from—
everything from meditation and Tantra to therapeutic bodywork practices. You'll
find a complete list of somatics resources in *The Survivor's Guide to Sex*.

What's it like to come back into your body? It's like awakening to a sense—
such as touch—you've read about, heard about, thought you understood, but
have never truly experienced.

You Are What You Eat

"Not treating your body as a temple can kill even the most Herculean libido,"
writes Heather Corinna in *Scarlet Letters*, her e-zine of femme erotica. "Healthy
sexual functioning requires a good respiratory system and a healthy flow of
oxygen, adequate hormone levels and properly functioning sexual glands, and
most of all, energy. The best diet for your sexual health is the best diet for your
health, period."[3]

Your body requires nutrition, adequate rest, plenty of fluids, and movement
to sustain life, much less thrive. You can improve your relationship with your
body by learning to take good care of yourself. In fact, tending to your physical
care is a great prelude to sex.

Get a Pelvic Exam

Add to this good health care. Many lesbians fail to get regular gynecological
exams, and even when we do get checkups, we're often not candid about our
sexual practices.

My ass! Definitely I like my ass!
I got a nice big old round booty that looks
good either in clothes or out.

Why don't lesbians get better health care? In the United States, lack of access to health insurance is a big factor in preventing women from getting adequate health care. Many lesbian and bisexual women as well as transgendered people feel very uncomfortable talking to health care practitioners about sex. (Many of us feel uncomfortable talking to our *lovers* about sex!) It doesn't help that few of us have access to health care professionals who have any idea what we *do* sexually. Some lesbians feel uneasy about the mechanics of Pap smears; others think that because they don't have sex with men, such care is unnecessary—not true!

Regular gynecological exams will help you stay on top of the state of your sexual health. Some sexually transmitted conditions don't produce noticeable symptoms until you've got a serious problem. For example, HPV, currently the most widespread sexually transmitted condition, has been linked to cervical cancer. A recent study conducted in Seattle found human papillomavirus (HPV) present among lesbians—even those who had never had sex with men.[4] A Pap smear can alert you to the presence of abnormal cells caused by HPV, long before cancer develops. However, you will need a complete gynecological exam, including blood work, to determine if you've been exposed to HIV or other STDs.

Safer Sex, Please

We hear a lot about safer sex—but what is it, really? Safer sex is the practice of assessing risks and taking precautions that you hope will prevent you from acquiring or transmitting STDs.

How do you know if you're at risk? Well, the greater the number of people with whom you have had unprotected sex, the greater the risk you've been exposed to a sexually transmitted disease. Your risk for acquiring an STD increases if you already have an STD, if you've used intravenous drugs, or if any of your partners have used intravenous drugs. Finally, some sexual activities are riskier than others (see "Safer-Sex Guidelines for Lesbian and Bisexual Women" below).

You may believe that because you're in a committed monogamous relationship you're exempt from safer-sex concerns. If that were true, there would be far fewer lesbians with herpes and HPV! Unfortunately, monogamy is *not* a foolproof safer-sex strategy. Some STDs can lie dormant for months or even years after exposure, which may be longer than your previous relationship. You could easily transmit an STD you didn't know you had. And, of course, a commitment to monogamy is no guarantee. Many women have sex outside of their relationships without telling their partners.

Here is a recommended safer-sex strategy for *monogamous* couples (two partners having sex exclusively with each other): For six months, use latex barriers every time you have sex (see the safer-sex techniques, below). After six months, both of you can get thorough gynecological exams, including a Pap smear and blood tests for STDs. If all tests are negative, you may decide to forego latex barriers. However, if one of you has a viral STD, such as herpes, HPV, hepatitis C, or HIV, safer-sex practices are recommended to prevent transmission of the STD. If one of you has a bacterial STD, such as chlamydia, use latex barriers until you've completed treatment.

Some women in *nonmonogamous* relationships choose to *fluid-bond* with their primary sexual partner. They share bodily fluids with only that partner, while using latex barriers with everyone else. Should one partner "slip" and engage in unsafe sex with an outside partner, the commitment is to tell the other right away. The partners can then assess the risk and make safer-sex decisions. Again, this presumes a high degree of trust.

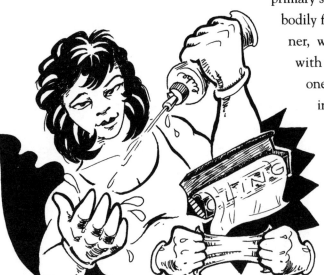

ILLUSTRATION 2. SAFER-SEX GEAR

Asking a new partner about her STD status is not foolproof either. While it's good to know a partner's story, you can hardly take a thorough sexual history on a first date. Even if you ask all the right questions and get all the right answers, you can't assume that a new acquaintance is being truthful—no matter how charming she is. She may have an STD and not know it.

Whether you have one partner or many, if you don't know your partners' sexual practices, health status, and sexual history—and *their* partners' practices, health status, and history—you'd do well to practice safer sex. Of course, if you don't know your own sexual health status (because you haven't been tested for HIV and other STDs), you need to practice safer sex to avoid transmitting an STD to your partners. And if you know you have an STD, then you need to practice safer sex.

Here are some basic techniques for safer sex between women. (See also Chapter 16, "Safer Sex and Gynecological Health.")

- *Oral sex:* Use dental dams, Lollyes, or plastic wrap for cunnilingus and rimming. Put a drop of water-based lube on the genital side of the dam. You can also cut up a latex glove or unlubed condom to make a barrier for oral sex (see illustration).

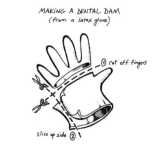

MAKING A DENTAL DAM
(from a latex glove)

① cut off fingers

slice up side ②

③ put tongue in thumb

ILLUSTRATION 3.

MAKING A DENTAL DAM

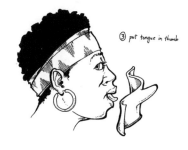

MAKING A DENTAL DAM
(from a condom)

① cut off top

slice up side ②

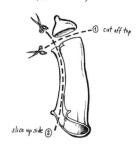

③ stretch!

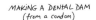

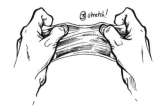

- *Finger fucking and fisting:* Use gloves for hand-to-vagina or hand-to-anus penetration.
- *Change gloves* when moving from anal to vaginal penetration and when you change partners. Remove the glove before you touch yourself.
- *Masturbation:* Don't touch your vulva, anus, or favorite sex toy with the same hand you've just used to touch your partner's vulva or anus—change hands or wash up first!
- *Dress your toys:* Use condoms on dildos, butt plugs, and vibrators.
- *Sharing toys:* If you share toys, be sure to use condoms and clean thoroughly between uses with an antibacterial soap.
- *Use water-based lube:* Never use oil-based lubricants with latex products (oil will break down latex).
- *Avoid products with nonoxynol-9:* While "noxious-9" has been shown to kill HIV in some laboratory tests, it can be irritating to vaginal and rectal tissue. Certain women experience vaginal infections after using nonoxynol-9. The product can actually increase the risk of HIV transmission by irritating the delicate rectal tissue, providing a direct route to the bloodstream.[5]
- *Yeast infections:* If your lube is giving you yeast or other infections, switch to a lube that doesn't list glycerin as an ingredient.
- *Bacterial vaginosis:* If your partner has a vaginal infection, see a gynecologist—and refrain from unprotected sex with your partner.
- *Urinary tract infections:* Urinating after penetrative sex can help prevent a urinary tract infection. Remember to drink plenty of water as well.
- *Do not share needles* whether for IV drug use, play piercing, permanent piercing, or tattooing.
- *Blood play:* Wear gloves during any activity that may bring you in contact with a partner's blood, such as piercing, cutting, or shaving. Be careful not to stick yourself. Dispose of sharps properly.
- *Dispose of gloves and condoms carefully:* Turn gloves and condoms inside out as you pull them off to prevent exposure to bodily fluids.
- *Clean your sex toys* with an antibacterial soap after every use.
- *Wash your hands* frequently with an antibacterial soap.

Safer-Sex Guidelines for Lesbian and Bisexual Women

These guidelines are intended to help you make choices about sex with women. There are no absolutes—an activity in the low-risk category can become high risk if you have a small cut on your hand or a sore in your mouth. HIV can be transmitted through contact with blood (including menstrual blood), vaginal fluids, semen, and breast milk. HPV and herpes can be transmitted through skin-to-skin contact. Hepatitis can be transmitted through contact with blood and feces.

High Risk
- Unprotected cunnilingus during menstruation
- Unprotected rimming
- Unprotected penis/anal intercourse
- Unprotected penis/vaginal intercourse
- Sharing sex toys (without a condom)
- Sharing needles

Risky
- Unprotected cunnilingus when a woman is not bleeding
- Vaginal or anal fisting without a glove
- Vaginal or anal finger fucking without a glove
- Unprotected fellatio (ejaculating in mouth is a higher risk than not)

Low Risk
- Cunnilingus with barrier
- Hand-to-vulva contact (no penetration)
- Vaginal or anal fisting with a glove
- Vaginal or anal finger fucking with a glove
- Fellatio with barrier
- Frottage (without clothes)
- French kissing (wet kissing)

Risk-free
- Frottage (with clothes)
- Nipple and breast stimulation (not lactating)
- Sharing sex toys (with a condom)
- Masturbation (only touching yourself)
- Voyeurism and exhibitionism
- Cybersex and phone sex
- Fantasy

Be Present

Sex is always more gratifying when you are *really there*. Not skin-deep, not hiding, not distracted, not anesthetized, and not suffocated under a molasses-thick blanket of shame—but fully available to engage in the moment. Whether you are flying solo, enjoying a sensual tangle with several partners, or gazing soulfully into the eyes of your one true love, it's good to be present for the experience.

Being present is the bottom line for most spiritual practices. Meditation, ritual, and prayer are all intended to bring the consciousness to the moment. What's this got to do with sex? Well, many people find a powerful connection between sex and spirituality. Tantra, essentially a spiritual tradition, has become the basis for sexual techniques designed to refocus erotic energy from "slam-bam-thank-you-Ma'am" to something a bit more, well, holy.

Others find sex to be a rare oasis of animal nature in our overscheduled, too-civilized urban lives. When else do we permit ourselves to loll in bed in the middle of the workday? An afternoon of sex will go a long way toward reminding you that you have a body—and a great capacity for pleasure!

On a more practical level, being present enables you to make meaningful choices about sex. This is what is meant by the term "consent," which Staci Haines defines as "the ability to choose, based on your own internal experience, what you want physically, emotionally, mentally, spiritually, and sexually, and then to communicate those wants."[6] How can you consent to sex if you don't have a clue about what you want—or even what you're feeling?

Being present for sex means not shutting down and not hiding the truth of who you are and what you want (or don't want). Being present means not bingeing, purging, or starving yourself, and not getting drunk or high to have sex.

I used alcohol as social lubricant so that I could get to the sex part. Now, though I'm not in recovery, I prefer to have sex sober, just because it increases the intensity for me.

Being fully available—in body and spirit—means dealing with problems that rob you of your life. There's no shortage of resources to help you become fully available for your life. Therapy, support groups, 12-step programs, and bodywork can help. See the "Resources" for more information.

I love the feeling of connection I get from making love with my girlfriend.

Life Changes

Even in bliss, when your dreams come true, your relationship to your body can be challenged by change. Pregnancy and childbirth, that longed-for breast reduction surgery, or beginning gender transition cause upheaval in your life.

Rachel Pepper, author of *The Ultimate Guide to Pregnancy for Lesbians*, reminds her readers of the importance of love and support to cushion the shock of change:

> *After spending so many years in the same body, it's disconcerting to watch it change so dramatically, so quickly.... As you go through physical changes, your partner can let you know you are still attractive to her. Many pregnant women get shy about their bodies when they start morphing. Of course, some partners know there's nothing more sexy than a pregnant woman. Those breasts! Those hips! That curvaceous belly! That growing life within! Your girlfriend can help boost your self-esteem by lavishing you with praise.* [7]

Many significant life changes happen *to* us, not *by* us. Crushing blows—such as the death of a loved one—can rock your world and with it your sense of comfort in your body. The end of a relationship can shake your self-confidence like almost nothing else. A severe illness or a sudden or chronic disability can sharply challenge your sense of self. Recovery from an eating disorder or addiction can toss you around on a roller-coaster of emotions. Menopause and aging can be both freeing and challenging to your sense of yourself as an erotic being.

You may feel that you can't be sexual while swimming through so much emotion. You may not want to get involved romantically just now. Perhaps you believe that fully experiencing your sexuality is disrespectful to a lost lover. You may feel very protective of your newly gendered body. You can take a break from erotic play—or a break from partner sex. This may be an opportunity to discover and pleasure yourself. Chapter 5, "Masturbation," will tell you how!

You deserve a fully satisfying sex life—all the pleasure you desire (in fact, all the pleasure you could ever imagine), on your own terms, without apology or price tags.

NOTES

1. Carol Queen, *Exhibitionism for the Shy* (Down There Press, 1995), 46.

2.   Staci Haines, *The Survivor's Guide to Sex* (Cleis Press, 1999), 16.

3. Heather Corinna, "Aphrodite's Appetite: The Ins and Outs of Eating for Great Sex," *Scarlet Letters*, May 1999.

4. Jeanne M. Marrazzo, Laura A. Koutsky, Kathleen L. Strine, et al., "Genital Human Papillomavirus Infection in Women Who Have Sex with Women," *Journal of Infectious Diseases*, vol. 178, 1604–609, 1999.

5. Tristan Taormino, *The Ultimate Guide to Anal Sex for Women* (Cleis Press, 1997), 36; Cathy Winks and Anne Semans, *The New Good Vibrations Guide to Sex* (Cleis Press, 1997), 73; and San Francisco Sex Information.

6. Haines, *Survivor's Guide*, 103.

7. Rachel Pepper, *The Ultimate Guide to Pregnancy for Lesbians*, 128.

chapter five

Masturbation

*Masturbation is fundamental
to my spiritual and sexual well-being.*

DO YOU MASTURBATE? When someone asks you what you like sexually, do you mention the ways in which you pleasure yourself?

Think of masturbation as the foundation for your entire sexuality. Masturbation is how you learn what you like and how you like it. How much of yourself do you bring to the task?

A lot of us don't admit to ever masturbating. We get so many messages about the second-class status of masturbation—or, for that matter, of being single. Well, not so! Masturbation is a form of sexual expression like any other, no more or less "legitimate" than oral sex or strap-on penetration. So what are the myths you've heard about masturbation? Are you afraid that if you masturbate you'll become antisocial or vibrator addicted? That you'll hurt your lover's feelings when she finds out what hot sex you're having all by yourself? Do you think that if you stay home on Saturday night to masturbate you're a loser? Or a sex-crazed pervert?

Well, let me give you some good reasons to masturbate.

10 Myths About Masturbation

1. *Masturbation isn't real sex. Real sex is what you do with your girlfriend.* We were also told that sex is for making babies. Puhleeeze, let's not buy into this. Pleasure is as good a reason as any to have sex, and pleasuring yourself is as valid an expression of your sexuality as any other.

2. *If you masturbate too much, you'll grow hair on your palms—or your labia will get really big.* Or change colors. Or look weird. Not true! One look at *Femalia*, a collection of color photos of women's genitals, and you'll see that vulvas come in all sizes, shapes, and colors. (And no one has ever gotten hairy palms from self-pleasure.)

3. *People in relationships don't masturbate. Or they masturbate only when the girlfriend's out of town.* The corollary to this is: *Women in healthy relationships don't masturbate; if you have to do for yourself, you must be suffering from Lesbian Bed Death.* The opposite is more likely to be true: if you masturbate—filling your life with erotic richness—you probably won't suffer from lack of libido. And if you share your erotic energy with your girlfriend, maybe she'll get turned on, too!

4. *Save it for your girlfriend. If you masturbate, you're taking something away from your partner.* That's fine if your honey is your erotic twin. But what if your desires don't perfectly match on a 24/7 basis? Masturbation isn't being "unfaithful." The idea that your lover should satisfy all your needs—sexual, emotional, spiritual—not only is unrealistic, it doesn't leave much room for you to be *you*.

5. *If you masturbate you'll get addicted and be unable to have orgasms any other way. You'll become antisocial.* "I was far more antisocial when I was love addicted," writes Betty Dodson.[1]

6. *Masturbation is a lonely occupation.* Yes, masturbation can evoke loneliness, sadness, grief—as well as joy, excitement, and the feeling that you might burst with pleasure. Sex is an emotional experience, whether you're sharing that experience with a partner or flying solo.

7. *Masturbation is something you should do in private.* Some of us had "enlightened" parents. Instead of slapping our hands when they caught us masturbating, they told us it was OK—just don't ever let anyone see us doing it! No wonder we find masturbating for an audience so deliciously naughty!

8. *Women who jerk off too much are sex obsessed.* How much is "too much"? How much pleasure are you willing to allow yourself? A thimble full? A bathtub? An ocean?

9. *Autoeroticism is kinky.* It's "normal" to get off now and then, but dressing up, playing with toys, watching yourself in the mirror, and licking the juices from your fingers—that's kinky. Give yourself permission to touch yourself, look at yourself, smell yourself, taste yourself. (If it helps to think of yourself as the perviest girl on your block, go for it!)

10. *If you masturbate, you'll become very demanding, expecting lots of orgasms and a life filled with erotic delight.* Yes! Good for you!

What Will Masturbation Do for You?

You get to have pleasure…lots of it. You can get off, whenever you want. All this pleasure is for *you*—you don't have to worry about anyone else's desires or needs.

Relaxation, reduced stress, and a good night's sleep are all benefits of masturbation. And buzzing off is a much better reward than a candy bar for finishing that term paper or sending off that business proposal.

Masturbation allows you to experiment with new sexual activities in a safe setting. You can try new toys, new fantasies, even a new persona without embarrassment. You can experiment with extended orgasms, multiple orgasms, and ejaculation. You can get messy without worrying about offending a partner's aesthetics.

Masturbation is the key to sexual self-knowledge. You'll know what you like. How? Because you've tried it. You'll know what gets you off—not just that one trick you discovered at age 10, or that particular technique you learned from your last girlfriend. You'll discover a number of sexual activities, fantasies, and techniques that work for you.

> *Masturbating really taught me how to touch myself, and gave me a good idea of how to touch and stroke a lover—I know now, for instance, to slow my stroking of her clit when she's about to come, when she's nearing the loudest part of her orgasm, to prolong the most intense, delightful part.*

All that self-knowledge leads to self-confidence and sexual autonomy. You know you can take care of yourself. You know what gets you off; you'll have specific information to convey to partners ("What do you like?" "Oh, everything, I guess.").

You can't be intimate with others until you can be intimate with yourself. How well do you tolerate your own company? What kind of solo-sex partner are you? Through masturbation, you can develop an erotic relationship with yourself.

Think of masturbation as a way to practice self-love. Sure, it's easy to say you love yourself, but do you *act* on that love? Masturbation is part of self-care, as much as regular massages, gynecological exams, or trips to the spa. Here's a way to pour energy *into* yourself, even as the world pulls so much energy out of you.

Intimacy—closeness to yourself in times of solitude or closeness to others in moments of sharing and connecting— reflects your inner world as almost nothing else does. And intimacy begins from the inside; it begins with your own self.

STEPHANIE DOWRICK

And, while we're talking about self-love, let's not forget that your body is a very big part of your "self." Through masturbation you can learn to love your physical self.

Sex-positivity means accepting, supporting, and celebrating human sexuality in all its splendid variety. Why not begin at home by accepting your sexuality, your body, the things you like, the ways you respond to your own touch and your own imagination? You're never too old, too boring, too fat, too thin, too stressed out, or too timid to deserve a great sex life.

The Masturbation Workshop Adventure

It's no coincidence that the best sex educators teach masturbation as the basic tool to helping women expand their sexual possibilities. And masturbation is the one tool you're always packing! From *The Ultimate Guide to Anal Sex for Women* to *Exhibitionism for the Shy* and *The Survivor's Guide to Sex*, sex guides are filled with encouragement and advice about masturbation.

Sex-toy salespeople are cheerleaders for the power of masturbation. "You would be hard-pressed to find a group of people more enthusiastic about masturbation than the employees of Good Vibrations," write Cathy Winks and Anne Semans in *The New Good Vibrations Guide to Sex*. "Every time we talk to a customer about sex toys we're inwardly cheering, 'Go home! Masturbate! You can do it! You'll love it, we promise!'" [2]

Sex-ed pros like Betty Dodson, Annie Sprinkle, Carol Queen, Tristan Taormino, and others facilitate hands-on workshops designed to help participants become more sexually confident. Some teach particular skills, such as G-spot ejaculation,

Time Out!

Do you ever feel like your insides have shattered into a million pieces? Or that if you have to endure one more breakup you swear you'll give up girls forever? Time to take a break, sister!

Lots of people choose periods of celibacy, which is as legitimate a sexual choice as any other. For some, celibacy means not being sexual with others. For others, celibacy may also mean not being sexual with oneself. Both are fine options.

For some, taking a break from partner sex is a spiritual tool, a way to achieve a heightened awareness of one's own energies and place in the universe. For others, it's a strategy for coping with difficult life changes—a breakup, newly won sobriety, the death of a close friend, or the turbulence of recovery from sexual abuse.

But what if it's your partner who has taken time out from sex—though you're still interested in pursuing your desires? This can be very challenging—especially if you've made a commitment to be sexually monogamous with your partner. While you might not have chosen the circumstances, you may be facing a prime opportunity to learn more about your own sexuality: just you and your imagination, a loving dance for one.

When you take a break from exchanging sexual energy with others, all that energy is left for you. A break from partner sex can really move you forward and help you focus—you can finish that last semester of grad school or figure out what you want to do with your life.

Without the distractions of another person, you get to feel *all* of you. As Staci Haines writes in *The Survivor's Guide to Sex*, "Intimacy with yourself means accompanying yourself through all of your feelings, sensations, thoughts, wackiness, and imperfections."[3] That can be scary. Prepare to feel, really feel who you are from the inside, perhaps for the first time.

Most importantly, a period of celibacy is a choice. I'm not talking about those times when there's no one out there you'd want to hook up with; I'm talking about taking a break by choice. Nothing like choosing *not* to have sex to remind you that *all* sexual expression is about choice.

You're hot, you're wonderful, you deserve every sexual gratification life has to offer. Taking a break from romance can help you to enrich your relationship with yourself.

---

anal penetration, Tantric sexual practices, or the art of the striptease. All of them endorse masturbation as their core curriculum. Those who've devoted themselves to teaching others know that self-exploration is the key to sexual discovery.

If you had the opportunity to attend a masturbation workshop, what would you like to learn? Would you wish to change some aspect of your masturbation practice? Would you want to devote more time and energy to thoroughly pleasuring yourself? Would you want to figure out how to get out of a rut—try a new position, a new toy, or a new style of stimulation?

Tristan Taormino got just that opportunity. Writing for *On Our Backs*, Tristan reported on her solo session with Betty Dodson, the "mother of masturbation." Intrepid journalist that she is, Tristan arranged a private lesson. "I was so excited about this adventure I nearly peed in my pants," she reported. "I was going to touch myself for Dr. Betty Dodson!"[4]

Like any responsible Ph.D., Betty began the session by taking a client history—in this case, talking to Tristan about her masturbation habits and practices. "I've been jerking off since I was four years old, so I was pretty comfortable with it, but I still believed that I could benefit from Betty's expertise. You can never be too rich or too sexually skilled." Confessing her citizenship in the Prozac nation, Tristan told Betty that she'd had difficulty reaching orgasm lately and would like to try coming on her back, rather than her tried-and-true method of lying on her stomach.

Betty led Tristan through a genital self-examination in which she praised Tristan's shaved cunt, coached her as she began to touch herself, and offered up a basket of toys for Tristan's edification, including a Crystal Wand (the S-shaped Lucite dildo designed for G-spot stimulation), a Hitachi Magic Wand, and a barbell that resembles the Kegelcisor, designed by Betty herself.

So what happened? Tristan earned an A+ in pelvic thrusting, but got a big "needs improvement" in the breathing department. Betty also pointed out that Tristan's reliance on extreme direct clitoral pressure was self-limiting; if she could train herself to respond to other forms of stimulation, Tristan would be a more "versatile" lover. Apparently, even the *On Our Backs* Adventure Girl could learn some new tricks!

Tristan summed up the most important lesson of all: "Betty helped me remember something I knew, but sometimes tend to forget, especially when having really good sex with an amazing lover: the one person who holds the key to my pleasure is me."

You don't have to wait for an invitation from Dr. Dodson to brush up on your sexual skills. You can sign up for a hands-on sex workshop at the nearest woman-owned sex-toy store. Even if you don't have access to a sexuality workshop, class, or sex coach, you can rent an instructional video, like Fanny Fatale's *How to Female*

Ejaculate, in which a circle of women masturbate to ejaculation and orgasm, or Betty Dodson's *Celebrating Orgasm*, which offers a glimpse of Dodson's famous hands-on coaching techniques. (One sex-toy saleswoman calls this genre the "Jack La Lanne of lesbian porn"—because you can follow along with the exercises at home.)

Of course, you can schedule your own masturbation workshop-for-one, anytime you please. You can even set educational goals. Maybe you've never masturbated to porn. Now you can rent a video, unzip your jeans, and find out what it's all about.

Your workshop curriculum can focus on breathing, making noise, moving your legs, or not stopping after the first orgasm. Perhaps you've never had an orgasm—or you don't *think* you've ever had one.... This is your chance. What would you like to learn?

Teach Yourself Some New Tricks

I'm a traditional girl: I usually just stimulate my clit with my finger. Every once in a while, when I'm feeling particularly naughty, I enjoy penetration during masturbation.

We have all different ways of masturbating. Most women reach orgasm by stimulating the clitoris—either directly or indirectly. Whether you lie on your stomach and rock your pelvis into the palm of your hand or against the edge of your kitchen table, rhythmically squeeze your legs together, thrust a dildo into your vagina or anus, touch your clit with your fingers, or buzz off with your trusty Hitachi Magic Wand, you've probably discovered a way to masturbate that works for you.

I masturbate in bed on my stomach with both hands, using my sheet or some piece of cloth for friction. I've been masturbating that way for most of my life. I like to be leisurely about it—take a long time to fantasize and get turned-on, then sleep or rest for a while afterward.

For many women, childhood masturbatory discoveries are today's modus operandi. If at 12 you discovered you could orgasm by rapidly caressing your clit in small intense circles, you may still be masturbating that way. That's great—you've no doubt given yourself years of pleasure. But, like any great lover who gets into a rut, you can become predictable and boring.

Some of your masturbation techniques may be necessary for you to reach orgasm, such as a particular quality of stimulation, and some, such as a particular position, may be mere habit. Can you reach orgasm standing up—or do you have to be able to stretch your legs and curl your toes? What about clitoral stimulation? If the vibrator is held just below your clit, rather than nestled beside your left labia, can you still come?

You can train yourself to respond to different kinds of stimulation and different circumstances. The key is to be open to new possibilities and to be willing to suffer a bit of frustration in the interest of experimentation. OK, so you could play with that dildo for days and *never* have an orgasm. Forget about whether or not you're getting off, and just note the sensations. Can you feel the muscles in your vagina fluttering as you push the dildo inside you? What do you notice in your ass, legs, and feet? Follow the sensations as they course through your body. You may surprise yourself and reach orgasm from stimulation you never thought could take you over the edge.

> *I lie on my stomach with my knees slightly propping my ass in the air; I use my fist, with my thumb rubbing my clit; I rub faster and faster, sometimes stroking the clit or reaching to my vaginal opening and use my body weight as pressure.*

How-to's of Masturbation

Here are some favorite masturbation techniques:

- Treat yourself to ample time and privacy. Light some candles and put on music that arouses or soothes you.
- Lavish yourself with your most appreciative gaze. Get out the mirror. Spread your labia. With your finger, trace the parts of your genitals: labia, clit, vagina, perineum, anus. Feel the different textures of skin. Note the different colors.

- Caress yourself. Touch your breasts, belly, thighs, feet.
- Suck your fingers—or a nipple if your breasts are large enough to reach your mouth.
- You can lie on your back or your belly, sit in a chair, kneel or squat over your hand or dildo, or rub up against a piece of furniture.
- Run your fingers lightly over your vulva. Notice which areas have the most heat for you.
- Reach inside your vagina and draw out your lubrication.
- Even if you're quite wet, put some water-based lube on your finger.
- Draw your finger up from your vagina to your clit.
- Stroke and pinch your nipples with the same rhythm you use on your clit.
- Gently hold the shaft of your clit between thumb and forefinger; stroke the shaft and hood with your fingertip.
- If you like intense nipple stimulation, try a pair of nipple clamps—just remember that the sensation greatly intensifies when you pull them off!
- You can masturbate in the shower or tub with a hand-held shower attachment. Remove the shower head attachment and put your finger over the end of the hose to create a high-pressure stream of water. (Do not spray water directly into the vagina.)
- Tug on your clit or labia piercing.
- Circle your clit with rapid, intense touches.
- Slip two fingers into your vagina and thrust against your G-spot; with the other hand, press down on your pubic bone and mons—so that you're stimulating your G-spot both inside and out.
- Slip a finger, butt plug, or string of anal beads into your butt. (Do not use the same finger or toy in your vagina, to avoid a bacterial infection.)
- You can hold a vibrator against your clit as you penetrate yourself with your fingers or dildo, or you can thrust a vibrating dildo in and out of your vagina as you touch your clit.
- Rock your pelvis, move your legs.
- Breathe. Breathe. Breathe. Breathe into your chest, belly, and cunt.
- Make noise!

Solo Toys

There are lots of toys you can play with by yourself. Favorite among them are vibrators and dildos. You can play with nipple clamps, butt plugs, anal beads, and many items found in the produce aisle of your local grocery store. If you play with vegetables, make sure to wash them first—or use a condom. The same caution applies to dildos, especially if you like both anal and vaginal penetration; just change condoms when you change activities, or have fresh sex toys at the ready. And don't forget the lube!

> *I used carrots a couple of times but they're too cold, and I found out if you microwave them they're too soft!*

Some women manage elaborate solo rope bondage. (Do *not* asphyxiate yourself!) You can loop string through your piercings and link nipples to labia—which will create an interesting tension when you rock your hips! You can attach clamps or clothespins to the outer labia and inner thighs, tease yourself sensually with ice cubes or hot wax, and even do play piercing. You'll find more about sex toys and supplies in Chapter 15.

Erotica and Fantasy

Of course, your imagination can be the most wonderful sex toy of all. And erotica is a great fantasy stimulator. Whether you begin your masturbation session with some one-handed reading, a favorite video or audiotape, a lascivious phone call to a gal-pal, a visit to a sexy web site or online chat room, as you close your eyes to ride that delicious wave of pleasure, all sorts of surprising images may pop into your head. While you started out fantasizing about Pepper and Nina Hartley in *Suburban Dykes*, suddenly you morph into both the straight guy in the library stacks and the sadistic librarian who leads him on. Who knows? You could be the uptown housewife seduced by her butch plumber. Let your clit lead the way. Don't try to have the "right" fantasies— follow the images that get you wet. Exactly what kind of touch are you really craving?

How-to's of Orgasm

Masturbation is a good way to learn how to orgasm—and all the experts from Lonnie Barbach to Betty Dodson will tell you it's much easier to learn how to give yourself an orgasm than to learn to come with a partner.

To summarize the best of the advice:

- *Give yourself permission.* Pleasure is important—as important as food or air. You're no less deserving of sustenance than any other living being.

- *Experiment.* Touch yourself in a variety of ways. Find out what feels good to you. "If you don't orgasm, that's OK—what's important is your discovery of what feels good. You can build on this the next time you masturbate," advise Cathy Winks and Anne Semans. [5]

- *Take your time.* It may take you an hour or longer to reach a level of arousal that can take you over the edge.

- *Breathe.* Breathing will oxygenate your blood and move energy through your entire body.

- *Make noise.* You can't hold your breath when you're moaning!

- *Move.* Rock your pelvis, move your legs. Notice the energy building as you move.

- *Use a vibrator.* Many women find the intense, reliable sensations of the vibrator are necessary to reach orgasm.

- *Use lube.* Put some water-based lube on the head of the vibrator, on your finger, and on your clit. Spread the lube around so that it coats your entire vulva.

- *Stop and start.* If you get frustrated, back off and let your sexual sensation slowly build up again. "Try not to get too fixated on the orgasm or else 'trying too hard' might kill your arousal," write Winks and Semans. [6]

- *Don't tense up.* Play with the tension in your body. As Staci Haines notes, "Most people think of orgasm as a tensing of the muscles, but the more you can relax, the better, since it can be difficult for the muscles to go from a very contracted state into an even more contracted state for orgasm." [7]

- *Practice.* Lonnie Barbach recommends that you set aside an hour a day, every day, for up to six weeks. [8]

- *Do your Kegels.* Annie Sprinkle writes: "Squeeze the pubococcygeus muscles (the muscles you squeeze to stop the flow of urine) on the exhale. These squeezes can actually stimulate the clitoris and G-spot, while pumping up energy throughout your entire body. In other words, inhale while filling your belly like a balloon, exhale and flatten your back while contracting the PC muscles."[9]

- *Feel your feelings.* Sexual feelings can stir up grief, anger, or fear. Backing off from sexual stimulation may make sense in the moment—but the cost is dear.

- *Get help.* There are many ways to approach your sexual healing. You can try somatic healing practices designed to help you heal trauma in your body. You can see a therapist to explore why you have a problem reaching orgasm. You can work with a sex therapist or surrogate. Or arrange a session with an orgasm coach.

- *Read a Sex Guide.* Aphrodite, the savvy online advice columnist at A Woman's Touch boutique, reveals that *she* learned to masturbate by reading *Our Bodies, Ourselves.*[10] Even sex goddesses had to learn *somewhere!* Investigate videos, books, and workshops. See the "Resources" for details.

Masturbating with a Partner

> *I absolutely love to be a witness to a lover enjoying her own body; it is such a beautiful personal intimacy. I've used masturbating to turn my partner on, too, which is really fun. It is very empowering to be openly appreciated and acknowledged and not shamed for masturbating.*

You might find nothing is more tantalizing than your partner parading her arousal in front of you, working herself up to a colossal orgasm as you sit helplessly stewing in your own juices.

When you masturbate in front of your partner, you're inviting her to witness you pouring loving energy into yourself. You give her evidence that you value your sexual pleasure. It's a sign of trust to allow someone to witness you in such an unguarded moment.

Masturbating to orgasm in front of my partner brings up a lot of my issues around self-acceptance. I feel self-conscious because the spotlight's entirely on me—I'm being watched. I worry that I look funny when I come.

Not only do you get to revel in your partner's gaze, you won't have to cope with the problem of the well-meaning (but clueless) partner who has no idea how you like your clitoris stroked. If the idea of explaining your preferences leaves you tongue-tied, you can rely on your freshman English teacher's favorite rule: Show, don't tell!

I don't think twice about having a wank in front of my partner. Especially if she's tied up.

You may discover the exhibitionist in you; and she may discover her inner voyeur. Every time you take a sexual risk, the possibility exists that you may widen and enhance your sexuality.

You can also touch yourself during partner sex. Sometimes it's just easier to take care of your own orgasm and leave your partner free to concentrate on other things—reaming your butt, filling your vagina with her fingers, wielding the G-Spotter, or sucking your nipples. Many women discover that they can come more reliably, more intensely, more easily when they touch themselves during partner sex. And when your partner is relieved of the job of "making" you come, she may be more creative, more assertive, more confident in pleasuring you.

If you come by your own hand (or vibrator), it still "counts." I discovered this sexual truth while watching a gay porn video at a queer film festival. As the star was being anally penetrated by his well-hung partner, he stimulated his penis. I was struck by the similarity to lesbian sex and the practice of touching one's clitoris while being penetrated by a woman partner. That the star brought himself to orgasm during partner sex was depicted as totally hot. The theater (packed to overflowing with gay men) was so quiet you could have heard a pin drop—or a zipper.

Notice how generously you treat yourself. Do you bring as much creativity to your own arousal as you would to your partners'? If you masturbate once a week, is that OK? Once a day? Three times a day? How much pleasure are *you* worth?

Suggested Web Links:

ASK APHRODITE

    www.a-womans-touch.com

BETTY DODSON'S HOME PAGE

    www.bettydodson.com

NOTES
1. Betty Dodson, *Sex for One: The Joy of Selfloving* (Crown, 1996), 95.
2. Cathy Winks and Anne Semans, *The New Good Vibrations Guide to Sex* (Cleis Press, 1997), 48.
3. Staci Haines, *The Survivor's Guide to Sex*, (Cleis Press, 1999), 221.
4. Tristan Taormino, Adventure Girl, "I Came on Prozac with Betty Dodson," *On Our Backs*, vol. 14, no. 2, 7, April/May 1999.
5. Winks and Semans, *New Good Vibrations Guide*, 59.
6. Ibid.
7. Haines, *Survivor's Guide*, 79.
8. Lonnie Barbach, Ph.D., *For Yourself: The Fulfillment of Female Sexuality* (Signet/Penguin, 1975), 94–95.
9. Annie Sprinkle, with Jwala, "How to Have Energy Orgasms," Annie Sprinkle home page, www.heck.com/annie
10. "Ask Aphrodite," A Woman's Touch, www.a-womans-touch.com/additions/Howto.txt

SOURCE OF QUOTE
Stephanie Dowrick, *Intimacy and Solitude* (W.W. Norton, 1995), 5.

chapter six

Communication and Finding Sex Partners

Where do I find sex partners? I go after them.

WHERE CAN YOU FIND SEX PARTNERS? Well, just about anywhere. At school, in sessions of academic conferences, at work, at a bar, at a dance club, at the gym, on the subway, at a sex party, in a women's studies class, in your queer youth group, at a 12-step meeting, at church or synagogue, while doing community activism, through introductions from friends, via ex-lovers (and even the occasional ex-husband), and of course over the Internet.

More specifically, you can meet sex partners while shopping for sex toys, at a Dyke March planning meeting, in line at the queer film festival, at the women's basketball playoffs, on parent/teacher night at your child's preschool, while marching in your local Pride parade, at the International Ms. Leather competition, at the Michigan Womyn's Music Festival, at Novice Night at your local S/M group, in your neighborhood queer bookstore, through your polyamorous lovers, and in the park while walking your dog!

Geography, Not Destiny

Whether you live in Louisville or London, the basics of meeting potential sex partners are the same. Sure, finding lovers becomes difficult when you can count the lesbians on your campus on your fingers—and still have a couple left over to vent your frustration! If your town boasts few queer social resources, you'll have to muster all your creativity (and self-confidence) to find sex partners. But even in cities with bustling queer communities—New York, London, Berlin, San Francisco, Los Angeles, Sydney—the well seems to run dry at times.

You can fly to San Francisco for the annual Pride parade, line up on Market Street with the cheering crowd half a million strong, and overhear an adorable pierced-and-tattooed dyke complain that she can't find a lover. Deprivation thinking will keep you, well, deprived. Honestly, if you think negatively enough, you'll discover a dyke shortage in P'town at the height of summer.

Want to find a girlfriend, trick, fuck buddy, or summer fling? Indulge yourself in every erotic delight at your disposal—especially your own erotic imagination and capacity for self-pleasure. Shine on yourself.

And in the meantime, here are a few pointers for finding sex partners:

- Know who you are and what you want.
- Take risks. So maybe you're not a party girl—but how many invitations have you turned down lately?
- Get out of your shell. Never been to a club? Dust off those dancing shoes.
- Throw a party.

Where did I find her?
She responded to an ad I placed. We went out
a couple of times, but the timing just wasn't right.
Four years later, she was working in my department.
Soon we were flirting, teasing, and trading
little notes. I felt like a teenager again.
Finally, I left her a note that said,
"I would really like to kiss you."

- Get involved in your community. You'll meet women who care about the same things you do.
- Let your friends know you're looking.
- Go to a sex party—even if you don't have a date. Take a friend.
- Place a personal ad in your local queer press, in an alternative weekly, or online.
- Learn how to talk about sex. There's more to finding sex partners than moving to a city with favorable demographics or buying a new black leather miniskirt—though you *will* look irresistible in the East Village. Before you rent the U-Haul or spend next week's paycheck, learn some basic communication skills. You'll be a more confident and competent partner— and you'll learn about yourself in the process.

Talk Talk Talk

I like it when she squeezes my nipples and talks dirty to me while I beat off. Very hot.

Many women enjoy talking about sex. It can be thrilling to be told in scrumptious detail how much a lover wants you—and to tell her exactly what you plan to do once you get your hands on her.

Desire—communicated in no uncertain terms—is a gift we give each other. Think of your tongue as a sex toy (not just for oral sex!) and of sex talk as foreplay. Your words can stoke the fires as effectively as kisses and caresses.

Some lesbians love to talk dirty. We whisper sensual promises into eager ears. We send salacious e-mails in the middle of the workday. We leave outrageously graphic notes in gym lockers, patent leather purses, billfolds, underwear drawers, and peeking out from the floor mat in the Honda—on the driver's side, of course. We have long, wet phone conversations. We spend days online cruising chat rooms for eloquent lovers. We make home movies. We tape ourselves having sex, and, as one woman relates, we hit the playback button again and again and again.

My lover and I recorded ourselves making love and we played it back one day, attempting to follow along with the rhythms of that particular "session." It started with my lover going down on me. I could hear myself in the recording wiggling around, the sheets crinkling underneath me, and the wetness my lover caused between my legs. I could hear her licking me, in the tape and in the moment, as if in stereo. Her moans were echoing through my head, my moans were echoing through my head. As my breath became quicker in the recording, so did it in real time. My lover was so wet that when she rose to kiss me, all of my fingers entered easily, and she rode my hand. I had just barely gotten my fist inside her when she came. I could hear myself beginning to climax in the tape. I was tight, waiting for her to come inside me with her cock. When she did, I felt my entire body shudder, sucking her in. I lost track of what was happening in the tape. All I could do was feel her inside me and listen to our breath. I have never come so hard as I did that night. It was beautiful.

Effective sexual communication is the single most-useful erotic skill you can bring to a lover. As Susie Bright says, "No lover is able to look into your eyes and figure out how you want to get fucked in the ass."[1] Sexual communication includes being able to articulate your desires, fantasies, history, limits, and concerns—and being able to listen without judgment to those of your partners.

Communication skills carry a big payoff: Your sex life improves dramatically as you gain fluency in the vocabulary of your own desires. When you can tell a partner what you want—in plain language—she'll be more likely to meet your needs. (One woman wrote, "I would love to be fucked up the ass on the hood of my sports car"— a simple enough request!) Your partner will be inspired by your forthright manner, too. Soon, she'll be telling you things she's never said aloud before.

Asking your partner what she likes will also improve your sex life. You'll find out exactly how she likes to be touched, which will make you a better lover. You needn't worry about coming off as inexperienced if you ask your lover how she likes her clitoris licked. Even if you've gone down on a hundred other women, you still don't know how *she* likes it. *Asking* is the mark of a sophisticated lover. It's a great way to get used to talking about desire, too. If you're too shy to open up a dialogue about your needs, start with hers. (Just don't forget to come back to you!)

Talking about sex won't ruin the mystery or spontaneity of your erotic encounters. The romantic myths that great sex "just happens" and that a skilled lover can intuit your needs are just that—myths.

Once you're open about your sexual practices and fantasies, you can stop wondering whether you're "normal." As soon as you start telling friends and lovers the scenarios that fuel your dreams, you'll find out that you are hardly unique. Many people share your fantasies. In fact, some of your friends may come up with turn-ons even more kinky than yours!

Folks in the BDSM community (bondage, dominance/submission, sadomasochism) have elevated sex talk to an art form. Among S/M aficionados, it's a common practice to negotiate before engaging in play, exploring each partner's desires, needs, limits, and safety concerns to find a common ground from which to proceed. Even experienced players negotiate prior to each new encounter—as do novices, for whom a single item on a checklist of possibilities can produce hours of wonder and anticipation. Intimate partners find that ongoing negotiation helps to keep their sex life fresh.

Negotiating a scene won't make it less exciting. For instance, you can discuss an abduction scene in great detail without ruining the surprise of the capture or the specific content of what will happen when your partner whisks you away. Negotiation between equals is what makes power-play emotionally safe—and what distinguishes it from real-world, nonconsensual power dynamics.

Negotiation is best handled in a nonsexual setting rather than in the heat of the moment. Take time to think about what you want from the encounter. You can discuss your hopes and desires, past sexual experiences, likes and dislikes, emotional needs and hot buttons, as well as your limits—the things you *don't* wish to do. This is a great time to talk about STDs and safer-sex practices, too. More on negotiation in Chapter 13, "Play Nice! (...or Else)."

What traits do sexperts look for in a partner? Expressiveness tops my list. In fact, many women seek out partners who are able to freely articulate their erotic desires. Why? When you talk with a new partner about what you are going to do, you reencounter your own sexuality through her eyes. Sex becomes new for you.

Finally, communication is how you practice consent. Even if you know what you want, you can't give (or withhold) consent without communicating it.

Tongue Tied?

Sexual communication isn't just for the chatty and the brave. Anyone can learn how to talk about sex—even a Recovering Shy Person like Carol Queen:

> *When I was (not so very much) younger, the idea of getting up before a crowd and attracting erotic attention would have sent me into a panic. In fact, I couldn't even imagine doing much of that sort of thing one-on-one. My idea of talking dirty was "I love you" or—really bold—"Oh, yes!"*
>
> *Since then I've been photographed naked, recorded (video and audio) having sex, and performed explicit sex shows. That I've done these things is not only evidence of my recovery, they're part of it.* [2]

Many of our inhibitions about sex talk are cultural. We're taught what's appropriate to say aloud and what's not. Especially for women, the bold expression of sexuality can carry a hefty price tag. *Slut* and *whore* may be words you've reclaimed as badges of honor, but in the right context they can still silence even the most fearless among us.

You may be afraid that at the core your sexuality just isn't good enough. That by putting your desires into words, you'll expose your basic inadequacy. That people will see how boring you are. Or how perverted. Or how tame. Or simply different.

Many of us have been taught that asking for what we want is selfish—and therefore bad. "Having full say about your own body does not mean disregarding others' feelings. It means that you have full say over *you*, while others have the same say over *their* bodies and sexuality," writes Staci Haines. [3]

Whether your goal is a career at the peep shows or to be able to tell your lover exactly how you want your breasts touched, you *can* learn to feel comfortable talking about sex. After all, you had to be taught to choke over those sexual words. You weren't born that way—think of a 3-year-old, happily reciting her new vocabulary words ("*poop!*") and dropping her pants for all the world to see.

Here are some suggestions to get you started:

- *Make a vocabulary list*. What words do you feel comfortable using to talk about sex? Is it *cunnilingus* or *oral sex* or *eating pussy* for you? *Butt fucking* or *anal intercourse*? What do you call the parts of your body?

- *Know yourself.* Nothing like information to give you confidence. Now's a good time to compose your own Yes/No/Maybe list. Take a second look at the "Erotic Play" list in Chapter 2, "Desire and Fantasy." Which of these activities do you like to engage in? Which might you like to try, perhaps under very specific circumstances? And which are you sure you're not interested in? Write "yes," "no," or "maybe" next to each item. Don't forget to record the date—when you discover your list a year from now, you may be charmed by your innocence!

- *Talk to yourself while masturbating.* That's how Carol Queen learned how to talk dirty. Start with grunts and moans and work up to your own erotic monologues. For an added challenge, record yourself masturbating and talking dirty and play it back.

- *Engage a friend in a conversation about her or his sex life.* You might want to pick someone who's also struggling to break free of sexual inhibitions. Go to a sexy poetry reading or film together. Talk about the experience afterward.

- *Find out how other people talk about sex.* Listen to porn on audiotape or CD-ROM (the "Herotica" series is a great choice—see the "Bibliography").

- *Treat yourself to an online chat* or an evening of phone sex.

- *Go to a play party* or other group event where people speak openly about sex.

- *Take a class.* Even if "Talking Dirty" isn't among the course offerings at your local sex boutique, you can polish your communication skills in nearly any workshop or lecture on sexuality. See "Where to Learn More," below.

Who Are You Looking For?

I am attracted to big bodies. Give me the soft, plush, easy-to-roll-into bodies. Mmmmm.

What are you looking for in a partner? Do you want a sex partner whose sexual interests match specific interests of yours? An experienced bondage top? A fisting bottom? Are looks important to you? Age? Cultural background?

"Oh, I just want someone nice" is a response that indicates you probably haven't given this much thought. Perhaps you know what you'd like in a partner, but don't think you really deserve someone that great. You may have been taught that it's wrong to objectify a potential partner by naming such specific preferences. If *you* don't own your preferences, someone else will do it for you. So take a pencil and paper, or call your best friend, and start a list of qualities you're looking for in a sex partner.

You can also get too specific for your own good. So, you're looking for a butch Latina dyke, 25–29, at least 5'8", strong build with voluptuous breasts and big hands, who works in the helping professions, enjoys softball and all-night poker games, Truffaut films and mystery novels, nonsmoking, kinky S/M top, who loves kids and dogs? Great. That's a start. But will you consider her if she's 34? Only 5'5"? Programs computers? Enjoys an occasional cigar? And hates gambling?

Give yourself permission to pursue sex—any kind of sex you can imagine on terms of your choosing. You don't have to pretend to romantic interests you don't feel. Likewise, you needn't pretend that you want to play when what you *really* want is to find a lover. Are you looking for a woman who will want only you? A polyamorous lover? A safer-sex buddy? Do you want to find a partner with whom you can break out of a rut? Are there particular sexual activities you want to try?

> *I've gotten better at asking for what I want and finding partners who like the same kind of sex I do. Being polyamorous, I frequently seek in one relationship the sex I'm not getting in another.*

Ask for what you want (not what you think you *should* want). You don't have to mold your desires to fit a political agenda. You needn't feel guilty that you are turned on by women of a certain body type or that you want to meet someone whose culture resonates with yours. You can always change your mind!

> *I went through this black-dykes-only phase. Looking back, I think of it as a cocooning phase. I was focused on learning about who I was in the world, coming into an understanding of my blackness, and I didn't want to be concerned with the needs or beliefs of white women. However, I did have a very powerful sexual*

reaction to one white woman. Eventually, I took this as an opportunity to explore the ways that my desire did not follow my politics. I had to find a way out of this discomfort, which was very much about boxing myself in. But it was also important for me to continue to make my beauty, my desires, and my culture the center of my world. Attraction for me would never equal loss of self or assimilation. Which is what I think I had feared.

Making Your Move

It's time to make your move. Now what? Surely there's more to sexual communication than lewd invitations whispered in a cloud of hormones. What about the thornier issues of partner sex? For instance, how do you ask someone to have sex with you?

Many of us have been taught to wait for someone else to make the first move. Have you ever convinced yourself that if *she* isn't making a move, she isn't interested? This would be comic if it wasn't so tragic—since she's probably thinking the very same thing. You have only one sure way to rise above misperception: Ask her. The trick is to ask in a context-appropriate manner. The statement "I find you extremely attractive, and I'd love to spend some time with you. Would you like to get together?" is acceptable in almost any situation. "I'd really like to touch you. May I?" is best saved for the dance floor or a sex party.

You can state the conditions under which you *might* like to have sex: "I'd love to play. But I'd like to get to know you a bit better first." You can check out a potential partner's relationship status: "I never date married women. Are you seeing anyone?"

You can invite a potential partner to engage in a particular activity and state your limits at the same time. "I'd love to play. But I'm not into penetration right now. Would you like to trade massages?"

You can trade interests, experiences, and fantasies—and get your message across quite clearly: "I hear you're quite a skilled top. I find the thought of submission quite tantalizing, though I've only bottomed once. Would you be interested in showing me the ropes?"

"No, Thank You"

Of course, sometimes you get turned down. My own fear of rejection shrank to a manageable size the day I overheard a stunning femme graciously deflect a sexual come-on. The would-be suitor approached the femme and said, "We've been eyeing each other all day. I want you to know I find you very attractive." The femme responded, "Thank you." Period. She did not find it necessary to qualify her response ("Thanks, but I'm not interested in taking this further"), nor did she find it necessary to behave defensively ("No way!").

I understood in that moment that a genuine expression of desire had value, regardless of the response. I was no less beautiful or worthy a human being because someone said, "No, thank you." (I also understood that I needn't fear a rude or unkind response—since that would reflect a lack of grace on the part of the speaker, and say nothing about me.)

"No" is an expression of a preference and is as valid a response to a sexual request as "yes"—though it's not what you hope to hear. Respect that preference. Being told "no" is not an invitation to argue or persuade. Move on and ask someone else.

What if someone approaches you for sex, and you're not interested or available? If you like, you can say, "I'm flattered you asked, but no" or "Not right now, but check in with me another time" (if you really think you might be interested later). However, a simple "No, thank you" is enough. You don't owe an explanation.

Personal Ads

The world of personal ads offers a wonderful opportunity to practice asking for what you want. Personal ads are especially helpful if asking for sex face to face makes you feel shy.

Even if you have no intention of placing an ad, writing one is a useful exercise. Why? A good ad lists both the qualities of the person you're seeking and the qualities you have to offer—toss in a memorable headline, some vivid description, and a bit of witty repartee, all in 50 words or fewer. Not a small task even for a seasoned copywriter.

What's Your Style?

Monogamy:
Having sexual relations exclusively with one partner

Serial monogamy:
Engaging in a series of monogamous relationships, one after the other

Nonmonogamy:
Having sexual relations with more than one partner

Fluid-bonding:
A safer-sex strategy of using latex barriers and limiting sexual activities with all but a primary sexual partner

Polyamory:
Having sexual relations with more than one partner; some use this term to mean having more than one lover at a time

---

Check out the ads in your local queer newspaper or arts and culture weekly. The nature and tone of the ads will give you an idea of who's using this particular venue and what they're looking for.

Usually placing an ad is free, while those answering the ads are paying for the service. Often newspaper ads list a 900 telephone number (with rates as high as $3 per minute). Similarly, many Internet personal ad services permit users to post ads for free, while only site members can respond to ads. Membership fees vary. Commercial services such as America Online (AOL) offer free personals to members—essentially, these are bulletin boards where you can post an ad and often a photo. See the "Resources" for more information.

Internet

I found my current partner over the Internet. Risky? Yes. Silly? Perhaps. That aside, this is the healthiest, hottest, most solid relationship I've ever had.

Lately, women have been meeting and mating by way of the Internet in growing numbers. Whether or not you intend a face-to-face encounter, you'll find buzzing conversations, flirtations, and sex.

As a medium for meeting people the Internet has some advantages:

There's something for everyone on the Net. If you can imagine it, you can probably find it, and if not, you can start it.

You can transcend the limits of geography. Even if you feel isolated in "real" life—the only boy-dyke in your campus queer group, or the only lesbian in a wheelchair in the entire county—you can create your own virtual community.

Beauty isn't always skin deep, and while many women exchange photos online, many more get to know one another through conversation…which is something of an equalizer, as you don't need to have the latest "do" to attract attention. Net chats are great for those who feel more comfortable in conversation than on the dance floor.

There's safety in anonymity; you can ask questions and try new things without worrying about looking silly.

You can be anyone or anything you like. No one knows you came out two weeks ago. No one knows whether you're preop or postop online. You can grow accustomed to being *yourself* in the world.

One person's Internet advantage will be another's disadvantage. That written and conversational cues supersede visual and cultural cues isn't a selling point for everyone—not everyone feels comfortable communicating in writing or wants to learn how to use a computer. There's a lot of trite conversation on the Net. You have to put up with men harassing women in lesbian chat spaces, and spam, endless spam (bulk mail advertisements). And publicly accessible chat rooms can be infiltrated by queer bashers and trollers.

The same freedom of anonymity that allows you to change persona when the mood strikes allows others to manipulate and deceive. You have to be just as cautious in opening your heart on the Net as you do bellied up to the bar.

You may think all these references to the Net are frustrating for those not online, not computer savvy, or lacking any desire to traverse the alphabet soup of World Wide Web jargon.

But actually Internet access isn't that hard to come by—or that costly. Most public libraries have computers available to patrons, free. Of course anyone connected to a university has access. You don't have to rely on your corporate e-mail account—which might be a bit dicey, considering the mail you hope to find in your "in" box! However you get connected, you can sign up with Hotmail, Yahoo, Excite, and other gateway sites for a free e-mail account. At home with your PC or Mac, all you need is a computer modem and an Internet service provider (think of your ISP as analogous to the phone company—it provides the dial tone).

Internet resources include:

- Bulletin boards where users post messages on a variety of topics
- Live chat rooms
- Personal ads and matchmaker services
- E-mail discussion lists
- Usenet newsgroups (The original Internet discussion forums, newsgroups are similar to e-mail discussion lists—people post their views on a variety of topics. However, while only subscribers can post to most e-mail lists, newsgroups are open to anyone who wishes to download the daily posts or post their own messages. So groups like alt.sex.bondage are heavy with spam, attacks on women and queers, and off-topic posts.)

Talking Dirty on the Net

Many women first encounter live Internet chat on a commercial service whose user-friendly interface eliminates the need to learn complicated Internet software. Basically, when you open a chat-room file on AOL, an easy-to-use window appears. You can browse the names of all the other AOL members in the "room," read their real-time conversation as the messages scroll by, compose your own message, hit the Enter key, and jump in.

But AOL's terms of service (TOS) won't help you cozy up to those dirty words you were hoping to practice. Public chat rooms on AOL are staffed by attendants who will "TOS" you out if you get too graphic. AOL's policies are intended to prevent harassment and hate speech. Unfortunately, AOL prohibits *consensual* sexually explicit language right along with racial slurs and rude come-ons. For more information on AOL's rules, go to KEYWORD: TOS. For sexually explicit interactions, go "private"—by creating a private room (accessible only by invitation) or through instant messaging.

Many chat-room enthusiasts graduate from AOL to IRC (Internet relay chat), which Anne Semans and Cathy Winks liken to a high-tech party line.[4] Thousands of IRC "channels" feature explicit conversation on every imaginable topic.

The Woman's Guide to Sex on the Web by Anne Semans and Cathy Winks is the best resource available for those who are more comfortable learning from print resources. If you'd prefer to get your info online, you'll find helpful links at the end of this chapter.

Play Safe

Remember to exercise caution when meeting strangers—whether you make contact online or through a personal ad in your local paper. Talk on the phone before you make a date. Trust your instincts—if your gut says, "No way," don't go. You're under no obligation to follow through on an initial contact, though standards of etiquette still apply. (Call if you have to cancel a date.) Cafés are a great choice of meeting place for first dates with strangers—they're low-key, inexpensive, and public. Here are a few tips for safe play-dates with strangers:

- If possible, play at a sex club or party.
- Bring your own safer-sex supplies.
- Let your friends know where you'll be.
- Ask your date if you can give her phone number to a friend—a safe player will respect your caution.

Sex Parties

As Carol Queen so eloquently puts it, "Nice girls don't go sniffing like beasts around warehouses full of men with erect cocks and women decked out in lingerie and smelling of hot pussy."[5] Which is exactly what so many women love about play parties!

Play parties can be shadowy affairs in dungeons equipped with elaborate bondage stations, or sensual afternoon soirees with soft music and seasonal arrangements of fresh fruit. Parties tend to take on an individual flavor, and everyone has her favorites.

Sex parties, workshops, S/M demos, and other overtly sexual gatherings are prime places for meeting a new sex partner—or even a lover. The advantage of these events, of course, is that you can be sure to find someone who shares your particular sexual style—since talking about sex is encouraged, and cruising is often the whole point of the evening! More on sex parties in Chapter 14, "Play Parties and Public Sex."

Sex Talk Guidelines

How do you tell your hot new girlfriend her cunnilingus technique leaves a lot to be desired? How do you tell your lover of five years that you're dying to try out a new sexual technique, sex toy, or play partner? Before you enter couples counseling, try these basic pointers:

- *Emphasize the positive.* "I'd really like your tongue on the shaft of my clit. But I need firm, steady strokes to come—and *please* don't stop once I start moaning!" will yield a more positive result than "I *hate* when you change what you're doing just when I'm about to come!"
- *Be specific.* In her eagerness to please, "a little harder" might sound like an invitation to trade in her dildo for a jackhammer. How about 10 percent harder? 20 percent harder?
- *Be polite in turning down offers for sex.* A kindly spoken "No, thank you" is a perfectly adequate response. "What? Are you kidding?!?" will tarnish your karma.
- *Be polite in asking for sex.* Even if you've been living in bliss for a decade, your partner isn't required to put out for you. She's a human being, not a domestic resource. Say "please."
- *If you need it, ask for it.* Do you need lots cuddling after sex? Time alone? A protein shake?
- *Practice compromise.* This doesn't mean that you engage in sex you don't want—or that your partner should engage in sex she doesn't want. But sometimes it's fine to put your wants on the back burner. (Your wants, that is, not your needs.)

- *Ask her partner what she wants.* You can practice active listening by checking to make sure you heard her correctly. "So, are you saying that you really don't find nipple stimulation a turn-on?" Who knows? Maybe she just told you that she loves having her nipples sucked—but not until she's well-aroused.

- *Practice nonjudgmental listening.* As they say at the San Francisco Sex Information hotline, watch the "Ick!" response. You may not find her fantasies at all erotic, and you'd do well to turn down requests for sex acts that turn you off. But you don't have to make her sex "bad" just to say no to it.

- *Talk in a nonsexual setting.* It's easier to talk about sexual needs in a nonsexual context than in the heat of the moment. Grab a mug of tea and sit down at the kitchen table (unless, of course, that's where you're planning to have sex!).

- *Pick a time* when you and your partner are both relaxed and available. As she's running out the door, already late for work, isn't the time to tell her you want to change your sex life.

- *Don't compare* her to past lovers, put her down, or dump a long list of grievances.

- *Watch out for unspoken assumptions* and expectations: "If I can make you come, you'll never leave me."

Where to Learn More

Here's a tip for learning how to talk about sex: Attend a lecture or workshop on any specific sexual technique or form of sexual expression that interests you. While you're learning Advanced Oral Sex Techniques or How to Make Your Own Sex Toys, you'll be getting practice in hearing someone speak explicitly about a sexual practice—and you'll get practice sharing as well. You'll gain knowledge and confidence and feel less shy about telling your partners what you like.

No matter what the topic, most sex educators put communication at the top of their curriculum—since it's essential to partner sex. (Even a masturbation workshop will help you explore what you like, and knowing yourself is essential to effective communication.)

Signs of Healthy Boundaries

(Reprinted from Co-Dependents Anonymous)

- Appropriate trust

- Revealing a little of yourself at a time, then checking to see how the other person responds to your sharing

- Moving step by step into intimacy

- Considering compatibility before moving into a relationship

- Deciding whether a potential relationship will be good for you

- Touching only with permission

- Weighing the consequences before acting on sexual impulse

- Being sexual when you want to be sexual, concentrating on you own experience

- Maintaining personal values despite what others want

- Noticing when someone else displays inappropriate boundaries

- Saying no to unwanted food, drinks, gifts, touch, sex

- Respecting others—not taking advantage of someone's generosity

- Respecting self—not giving too much, hoping that someone will like you

- Not allowing someone to take advantage of your generosity

- Trusting your own decisions and accepting the consequences

- Knowing who you are and what you want

- Pursuing your own growth

- Recognizing that friends and partners are not mind-readers

- Clearly communicating your wants and needs [recognizing that you may be turned down, but you can ask]

- Talking to yourself with gentleness, humor, love, and respect

Many authors and other "sexperts" in the United States and Canada offer workshops and classes on specific sexual techniques. Staci Haines offers sexual healing workshops for survivors of child sexual abuse; both Tristan Taormino and Carol Queen offer anal sex workshops; Karlyn Lotney (aka Fairy Butch) teaches Dyke Sex: Power Tools, and other dyke sex classes; Annie Sprinkle conducts workshops on Tantra and genital massage; and Betty Dodson offers her famed masturbation workshops. While most of these women are based on either the East or West Coast, they do travel. The Michigan Womyn's Music Festival and other large national and regional gatherings are also great places to catch a traveling sexpert.

Sex-positive sex-toy boutiques often sponsor educational events. Sh! in London, Good Vibrations in San Francisco and Berkeley, Grand Opening in Boston, Toys in Babeland in both Seattle and New York City, A Woman's Touch in Madison, Good for Her in Toronto, and many other stores across the United States and Canada offer workshops and demos on everything from flirting to anal sex. Local S/M organizations frequently offer workshops and demonstrations— even if your interest in S/M is on the mild side, you may want to attend a program on negotiating with a new partner. See the "Resources" section for more info.

> *When I was 20 I had a girlfriend who was a total exhibitionist. She dressed to turn herself on, and turned on everybody she met. I learned my best-ever sexuality lesson: Assume that you—your body, your needs, wants, desires, and fantasies—are the hottest fucking thing on the planet.*

Suggested Web Links:

IRC HELP
>   www.irchelp.org

THE GUIDE TO LESBIAN CHAT
>   www.grrltalk.net

NOTES:
1. Susie Bright, *Susie Sexpert's Lesbian Sex World* (Cleis Press, 1990, 1998), 34.
2. Carol Queen, *Real Live Nude Girl: Chronicles of Sex-Positive Culture* (Cleis Press, 1997), 62.
3. Staci Haines, *The Survivor's Guide to Sex* (Cleis Press, 1999), 104.
4. Anne Semans and Cathy Winks, *The Woman's Guide to Sex on the Web* (HarperSan Francisco, 1999), 161.
5. Queen, *Real Live Nude Girl*, 68.

SOURCE OF QUOTE
"Signs of Healthy Boundaries" reprinted from a flier by Co-Dependents Anonymous.

chapter seven

Breast Play

I like it all—rough, gentle, caressing, grabbing, pinching, sucking.
Got the picture?

OUR BREASTS OFFER A DELICIOUS RANGE OF SENSATIONS. We enjoy caresses, fluttering kisses, moist lips on nipples. We like squeezing, pinching, kneading, slapping, and nibbling. We like having our nipples tugged and bitten, pulled and twisted. We enjoy soft touches around the curves. We crave feeling our breasts nestled together with those of a partner. We relish a woman's hands on our pectoral muscles. We luxuriate in voluptuous breasts overflowing our grasp and we adore pert breasts with pointed nipples teasing the palms of our hands. We delight in juicy bee-stung nipples that fill our mouths. We love hard masculine chests proudly fronting a woman's body. We even like to suck a drop of colostrom from a partner's nipple.

Breast play isn't only for partner sex. You can stimulate your breasts during masturbation—some women keep a set of nipple clamps by their bedside for just that purpose. Women with large breasts can even suck on their own nipples as they stimulate their clits.

Women who love breast play crave attention to their breasts, especially to the nipples. Their breasts seem to perk up at the possibility of touch, and once stimulated, they experience a current of sensation running from nipple to clit. Some women can reach orgasm from prolonged nipple stimulation alone.

As you get aroused, your nipples become erect and your aureola swells and may darken. Your breasts may seem to get larger. Like your clitoris, an aroused nipple maytake a *lot* of sensation. You may enjoy more intense nipple play as you approach orgasm. In fact, some women must be extremely aroused to enjoy any nipple play at all.

My nipples are extremely sensitive. I can't even wear clothing with seams there or bump against the edge of a table without feeling uncomfortable. So I have to be sexually stimulated before someone can touch them—but then I want it all, especially sucking—but not hard.

How women like their breasts and nipples touched is as individual as how they like their clits touched. It's not just a matter of whether you prefer light or hard touches, though that's important. You may be very particular about *how* you like your breasts touched. You may like the whole breast cupped and the underside caressed and held, or perhaps don't like the undersides touched at all. Experienced breast-play aficionados can get quite specific in their instructions for nipple stimulation.

I prefer delicate touches or licking around the nipple. Almost—but not quite—a tickling feeling. That's great! Love it!! Mmmmmm…

Sensitivity

Sometimes I'm very sensitive and just a gentle stroke will make me shiver or jump.

Breast sensitivity changes from day to day, over the course of your menstrual cycle, and over a lifetime. During your period, your breasts swell to their fullest and roundest—and may look quite succulent. Your breasts may be more sensitive in the days leading up to your period or during your period. Both PMS and pregnancy can make you feel as if you have "atomic tits."

New piercings, of course, will make your nipples especially tender. Fibroids can also make breast play painful. Any surgical procedure, such as a breast reduction or breast implants, can result in scar tissue that affects sensitivity. Of course, breast cancer will affect women very individually. Some women lose sensation after treatment, while others experience pain.

Two years after my lumpectomy, other people can hardly see the scar even when I point it out. I lost sensitivity in the nipple for a while but it's back almost full-strength now. I have ongoing irregular nerve pain inside the breast tissue around where the tumor was. Pressure directly on that area of the breast hurts like hell, so positions like lying on top take care. Sometimes if I mention this to a lover she or he seems scared and then avoids touching that breast. I understand but would prefer a more careful touch and inclusion of that breast in our sex play. I loved my breasts before, and I treasure them even more now.

Teach Your Partner

I never used to enjoy breast stimulation until I met my current partner. Perhaps no one had a soft or gentle enough touch for me...or maybe I just never allowed myself to feel what I've felt with her.

Breast play is an area where good communication skills can pay off. A delicate kiss on an oversensitive nipple can be pleasurable or excruciating—or both. Ask before caressing, sucking, pinching, biting, or using clamps or other toys. Don't assume that if you like light, subtle touches she'll like that, too—or even feel it! Or that if you like to have your chest mauled, your partner will as well.

I enjoy having my partner lick and suck and even nibble my nipples, but I think the thing I most enjoy is having the curves of my breasts caressed.

Next time you're in the mood to entertain your partner, show her exactly what you like. Let the exhibitionist in you run wild. Touch your breasts exactly as you would have her touch you. Then take your partner's hand in yours and show her what you want.

I like rough play with my nipples. I want to be tugged and sucked and bitten and pulled and twisted, and I want more and more and then some.

Just as important as showing your partners how your breasts feel is discussing how you feel about your breasts. You can't predict breast play preferences by breast size or even gender identification. How we feel about our breasts as objects of erotic attention is extremely personal. Just as not all femmes delight in breast worship, not all butches will retreat from a hand on their breast. However, they may be very particular about the kind of attention they receive.

I like my chest rubbed more than my nipples played with. I like it treated like a guy's chest.

Not all women eroticize their breasts. Many survivors of sexual abuse find the memory of it triggered by having their breasts touched. Which makes sense—if one's breasts were the site of unwanted, harmful attention. Some survivors skip breast play entirely; others guide their partners in how they can enjoy breast play.

How-To's of Breast Play

Here are some favorite breast play techniques:
- Lick your partner's chest and underarm, working your way to her breasts.
- Experiment with a range of sensations from very light touches to very rough.
- Lick and nibble the sensitive underside of her breasts.
- Bury your face between her breasts.
- Cup the breasts in your hands, squeezing them together.
- Press her breasts into your chest.
- Lick your fingers and swirl the wetness over her nipple. Or, use a drop of lube, edible flavored lotion, or even her own juices (if you don't intend to suck her nipple again or are fluid-bonded).
- Stroke her nipple quickly and lightly, alternating with sharp pinches.
- Blow on her moist nipple.
- Roll a nipple between your fingers. Lick and suck the tip as you would her clit.

- Squeeze her breasts together and lick both nipples simultaneously.
- Pinch and squeeze the nipples between thumb and forefinger.
- Grab a pair of nipple clamps to stimulate her breasts, leaving your hands free for other things.
- Rub your vulva over her breasts; or rub your nipple on her clit after orgasm.
- Turn a blow job into breast play. "Tit fucking" needn't be reserved for heterosexual porn. After she's sucked your strapped-on cock, slip your saliva-lubed cock between her breasts and thrust inside her cleavage. You can slide your cock back and forth between her breasts as she sucks.

Nipple Piercings

My piercings make my nipples one of my main sources of sexual pleasure. I can come from just nipple play.

Nipple piercings can make breast play even more deliciously erotic. Not only are the rings and barbells attractive and fun to play with, many women even find that their nipples become extra sensitive after they get piercings.

Nipple piercings can take several months to heal. New piercings can be quite raw. They're also vulnerable to infection. So, if you're playing with someone who has a piercing, make sure you ask how recently she got it. Ask your partner how her piercing affects nipple sensation, too—some women lose nipple sensitivity as a result of scar tissue forming at the point of entry.

*I like when she wakes me up
in the morning by suckling my nipple.
My lover can make me orgasm
just from stimulating my breasts.*

Toys for Breast Play

You may not ordinarily think of your clothes as sex toys, but lingerie and fetish wear are popular erotic playthings—especially for the exhibitionist. Delicate structures of lace that emphasize the shape of the breast, corsets that enhance cleavage, brassieres with holes where nipples can peek through, leather harnesses, and chain-mail halters—all are designed to draw the eye to your breasts.

Bondage enthusiasts can create elaborate corsets of rope as beautiful and alluring as any garment you can find. Breast bondage is especially fun with large-breasted women. Wrap thick, soft rope around each breast and then in a figure eight linking the breasts. All bondage safety precautions apply: *Do not* use thin wire or string that can cut, *do not* wrap rope tightly enough to cut off circulation, and *do* make sure you have safety scissors handy in case of emergency.

For sensual breast play, you can experiment with feather boas, fur mitts, battery-operated vibrators, light slappers, and soft whips. You can play with suction toys, such as tit pumps and snake-bite kits. You can create a range of sensations by altering skin temperature through the use of ice cubes, mentholated cough drops, Tiger's Balm, and hot wax. You can produce ecstatic (and/or excruciating) sensations with fingernails, feathers, slip-on talons, and even the neuro wheel your chiropractor uses to test your reflexes.

Nipple clamps are perhaps the most popular toy for breast play. Clamps come in a range of styles and intensity, from barely hugging the nipple to biting hard enough to leave teeth marks. Some are adjustable. Homemade substitutes for tit clamps include clothespins and clips you may find in an office supply store.

When my lover sucks and pulls my breasts,
I sometimes like to imagine that I'm
restrained by some kind of device that holds
my nipples as people explore my body.
God, I love that.

Examine the clasp or teeth of the clips—some are sharp enough to draw blood, so choose accordingly. Clamps can be placed directly on the nipple—which is very intense. You might want to experiment with new clamps on your *own* breasts to gauge their intensity. Pinch a small amount of skin on the side of the breast or even on the aureola—see how much sensation you like.

> *I like nipple clips. I like to wear them pretty tight for about ten minutes, have them taken off, and then have my nipples rubbed, licked, and sucked on.*

Clamps restrict the flow of blood to the pinched tissue. After a little while, the pinching sensation fades as the area goes numb. When the clamp is yanked off, blood rushes back into the area, waking up the nerves. No wonder that clamps hurt *more* when they come off than when they go on. (*Do not* leave clamps on for more than 20 to 30 minutes, to avoid damaging tissue.)

Many of the toys used in sensual breast play can be intensified for those who like true torture. The temperature of melted wax can be controlled by adjusting the distance of the candle from the body. Holding a burning candle inches from your partner's nipples will result in searing drops of wax. Temporary piercings with sterile needles will produce very intense sensations. Some women's breasts bruise very easily, which they may or may not like. Ask before you swing a cane or rubber flogger. For more information, see Chapter 13, "Play Nice! (...or Else)" and Chapter 15, "Sex Toys and Accoutrements."

chapter eight

Clitoral Play

*Her fingers are like magic wands that do crazy
things I didn't know were possible.*

MOST WOMEN NAME THE CLITORIS AS THE MOST EROTIC SPOT ON THEIR BODIES.
For those of us who rate clitoral stimulation as our favorite source of sexual
pleasure, no sexual encounter is complete without direct clitoral play.

*I love when she moistens the tip of her breast with my wetness and stimulates my
clit with the nipple.*

Clitoral play includes stimulation with fingers and hands, thighs, butts and
pelvis, erect nipples, tongues, and lips (see Chapter 9, "Oral Sex"), as well as
vibrators and other toys.

Clits come in all shapes and sizes and are as individual as the women who
own them. Your clitoris may be a tiny pearl hidden beneath the folds of its hood
or as big as a thumb protruding from your lips. It can be deep red, pale pink, or
dark purple—and the color will deepen with arousal. You may crave intense
clitoral stimulation or quiver at the slightest caress of a fingertip over your clitoral
hood.

Understanding that the clitoris is hardly the little "nub" described in
traditional anatomy texts will broaden your approach to clitoral play. The clitoris

is an extensive structure of erectile tissue, beginning at the top of the vulva with the body of the clitoris (glans, hood, and shaft), cradling the urethra, and reaching down to flank the vaginal opening. (See Chapter 3, "Anatomy and Sexual Response.") Stimulating the body of the clit is just the beginning. You can direct your attention to your partner's labia, urethral area, vaginal opening, and perineum. Of course, when she begs *"Please touch my clit!"* you can return your focus to her clitoral glans, hood, and shaft.

The Art of the Hand

Lesbians have sensitive hands—after all, we make love with our hands. We use our hands to caress and arouse our partners, and to bring them to orgasm. Many of us are very tactile; we get off from touching as much as from being touched. Through our hands, we ride our partners' pleasure.

However, the myth that every lesbian or bisexual woman innately knows how to touch another's clitoris is just that—yet another myth. Women are far too specific about our preferences for this to be true.

> *I like my clit touched low, down near my urethra, and rubbed around in a circle, like a ball.*

Traditional sex guides toss off touching as "mutual masturbation"—as if pleasure we deliver with our hands (and, for that matter, masturbation) doesn't count as "real" sex. Of course, *we* know better!

Take a Tour

There many ways to discover what kind of clitoral stimulation a partner will like, and the discovery can be equally fun with a new partner as with a partner of many years. For starters, ask her. In bed or at a café, you can initiate a conversation that may well be a prelude to hot sex.

You can request a tour of her vulva. If she has even a drop of exhibitionist tendencies, she'll be more than happy to oblige you. And if you have a hint of the voyeur in you, this could make an exciting sexual scene in itself.

Pick a time when you're both relaxed. Make sure the room is warm enough to be nude comfortably and well lit enough that you can see every fold and detail of her vulva. Ask your partner to undress—you can strip down as well. Arrange lube, gloves, and sex toys nearby.

Ask your partner to touch herself for you. Watch how she handles her labia and clitoris. Notice how many fingers she uses, and whether she focuses her touch on the left or right labia, the clitoral shaft or hood, under the clitoral glans, or directly on the glans itself.

Then, take your own tour. Begin by massaging her inner thighs, butt, and outer labia. Snap on latex gloves, add plenty of water-based lube, and open her lips. Notice the glans of her clitoris. Has it retreated in its hood? Is it erect? How big is it? Are her lips engorging under your gaze? What color are they? Do her inner labia protrude from the outer lips?

Our hands are our first sexual tools—stroking, squeezing, caressing, kneading, grabbing, tickling, pinching, and slapping. Although very little pornography celebrates hands, a connoisseur will look at a new partner's palms, fingers, and forearms, and evaluate the quality of their touch, and give it equal weight with the more obvious attributes.

PAT CALIFIA

Stimulate her entire vulva—outer labia, inner labia, perineum, the opening of the vagina—before you concentrate on the body of the clitoris. Run your fingers through her pubic hair, or, if she's shaved, stroke the silky bare skin of her outer labia. Ask her which of your caresses she likes best. Pay attention to her responses—both verbal and nonverbal.

Many women prefer indirect stimulation until they're extremely aroused. They may like caresses to the side or just above the clitoral glans. With arousal, the clitoris becomes erect and swollen and can take a lot more direct stimulation.

Your partner may like small circles traced lightly over the glans with just the tip of a forefinger, or a back-and-forth rubbing motion on the side of the clitoral shaft. She may like to feel two fingers sliding rapidly on either side of the clitoris. She may like you to press firmly on her mons with one hand as you stroke her clitoris with the other. Many women enjoy clitoral stimulation combined with vaginal or anal penetration.

Most woman require sustained stimulation to come. Some women reach orgasm best with increased speed and intensity; others prefer a very slow progression to orgasm, drawing out every last wave of sensation.

After orgasm, your partner may desire continued stimulation and may ride that coming into another orgasm, a series of multiple orgasms, or one long tsunami of pleasure. If she can't tolerate such intense sensation, but doesn't want to stop, back off. Slowly gather momentum. Subtle, indirect stimulation may work to get her up to that edge again.

What If Your Hand Gets Tired?

A tired hand may be a sign that you're trying too hard—or that your partner isn't aroused enough to reach orgasm. Is she turned on? Observe her body's cues—moans, rocking hips, breathing. If you begin your sex play with direct clitoral attention, her arousal may never catch up to your level of intensity. Make sure she's well aroused *before* you touch her clitoris.

"Please just caress me for a little while." Of course, she can let you know that she's not turned on enough to even think of reaching orgasm. And she can tell you what kind of stimulation she would prefer. Ask her what she needs to come.

Lube, lube, and more lube! A slippery, moist vulva will get aroused faster than a dry one. Her perception of wetness will make her feel sexy; her own juices will start flowing. Lube up your fingers before you touch her clitoris. Refresh the lube from time to time as it dries up.

Human sexual response isn't linear. We move from arousal to plateau and back to excitement again and again before orgasm. Do you need to focus on orgasm right now? If your attentions are taking her nowhere, back off and build up again. Touch her in a spirit of exploration. Approach and back off over and over again to increase her arousal.

Combine direct clitoral stimulation with vaginal or anal penetration, rimming, nipple play, or other stimulation.

Invite her to touch herself or to guide your hand. Ask her to put your fingers in the right spot, and to show you the right pressure and rhythm. Lube up both your hand and hers, entwine your fingers, and let her take you both over the edge.

Grab a vibrator. You can hold a vibrator to her clitoris or put it in her hand. You can stimulate her nipples or penetrate her vaginally or anally as she uses the vibrator to reach orgasm.

Some positions are better than others for sustaining clitoral stimulation. With your partner on her back, sit facing her with your pelvis close to her hip and your hand between her legs. You can toss one leg over hers, bringing your pelvis close to her thigh. Besides closeness, the advantage of this position is that your wrist is lower than your elbow, reducing stress on your wrist and hand.

What if you simply can't sustain the action she requires? Conditions such as carpal tunnel and other repetitive stress injuries (RSI), arthritis, multiple sclerosis (MS), and other disabilities can limit your ability to use your hands as sex toys. Negotiate your needs. You and your partner can find activities that are gratifying—and pain-free—for both of you. Ask her to describe what kinds of stimulation she needs to get off. Describe your physical limitations, and tell her what kinds of sexual activities are comfortable for you. (Don't forget to tell her which ones you find especially hot!)

If you can't sustain stimulation with your fingers, and if using a vibrator aggravates your RSI, you can combine hand stimulation with other forms of stimulation. You can use your lips and tongue to supplement your hand. You can stimulate her nipples, tongue her anus, or bury your fist inside her vagina as she brings herself to orgasm. See "Sex and Disability: Toy Accessibility" in Chapter 15 ("Sex Toys and Accoutrements") for suggestions on selecting toys that will work for you.

Frottage

I can come by rubbing myself against my lover's body—especially if I've really got the hots for her.

Frottage (also called *tribadism* and *dry humping*) comes from the French verb *to rub*. Frottage involves rubbing bodies together to produce heat and friction. You can hump a partner's thigh, rub vulva to pubic bone, or vulva to tailbone. Lying on your belly, you can squeeze your partner's clitoris and labia between your ass cheeks; she can reach around, slip a hand between your legs, and stimulate your clitoris as she humps you.

Women with extremely responsive clits speak highly of frottage as a method of indirect stimulation. Those who prefer more direct sensation can add a vibrator to frottage. You can slip a wand-style electric vibrator between you. Or you can strap on a Leather Butterfly harness with an egg vibrator in its pouch. You can also combine frottage with stimulation from nipple clamps, butt plugs, and other toys.

How-to's of Clitoral Stimulation

Here are some favorite techniques for clitoral stimulation:

- Caress and nibble her inner thighs.
- Rub your thigh between her legs.
- Tease her clitoris with your nipples.
- Cup her vulva in your palm, feeling her heat.
- Grab a glove; thoroughly coat your fingers with water-based lube.
- Pull open her lips and caress her labia.
- Blow gently on the body of the clitoris (*do not* blow directly into the vagina).
- Let her anticipate your touch. Let her experience her own wanting. Don't poke directly at the glans or immediately dive for her clitoris (unless, of course, that's what she likes!).
- Start with a long, languid stroke from perineum to clitoris (take care not to draw bacteria from anus to vagina).

- If she says, "I'm too sensitive," switch to an indirect touch.
- Gently stroke the shaft of her clitoris. Let the hood protect the glans until she's well aroused.
- As she becomes more aroused, swirl your finger around her clitoral glans; stroke the glans with tighter and faster circles.
- You can nestle her clitoris between the forefingers of both hands, stroking rapidly on either side of her shaft.
- You can combine stimulation from your fingers with her favorite vibrator. Try holding the vibrator slightly to the side to give her indirect stimulation as you stroke her clitoris. Vibration on piercings can produce interesting sensations.
- If she has a genital piercing, you can thread a piece of brightly colored ribbon through the ring and give her the ends to hold or tug on.
- You can combine clitoral stimulation with penetration—either vaginal or anal or both. You can add a dildo, butt plug, anal beads, or insertable vibrator.

Genital Piercings

The first time a lover touched my new clit hood piercing, I almost could not deal with the tremendous energy surge in my body—as metal conducts electricity, so does it conduct lust.

Genital piercings can be quite functional—they can increase clitoral sensitivity and can be great fun to play with. Female genital piercings include clitoral hood piercings, triangle piercings (which pierce the tissue under the clitoral shaft), perineum piercings, and labia piercings—among others. Piercings can take from one to six months to heal, depending on the location and type of piercing. So it's

I celebrated my cunt with the most expensive piece of jewelry I own!

important to ask your partner how recently she got her piercing, if the area is still tender, and whether she's comfortable having the jewelry played with.

Clitoral hood and triangle piercings may place a bead right over the glans—which can make stimulation hugely exciting. Your thigh nestled in your partner's crotch can slide the ring back and forth over her clitoris. A vibrator touching the metal can make her jump. Some women like light slaps over the piercing—think of the little ring and bead ricocheting off her glans. Try holding a tuning fork to a partner's hood piercing—the vibrations of sound will go right through her clitoris.

Labia piercings *beg* for attention—they can be used for light bondage (do *not* use a piercing as a stress point for serious bondage, however). You can adorn her piercings with colored ribbons and even hang bells from them—you can hear her come in an entirely new way!

Genital Shaving

Shaving has always been a part of my sex life. There is more sensation and I love the closeness.

Many women love the look and feel of a freshly shaved pubic area. Shaving makes the entire vulva more sensitive. You may find that you respond to the slightest touch, even the caress of loose clothing. Many lesbians like the look of naked accessibility; they like to see the inner labia protruding from the outer lips.

There's nothing quite like the smooth skin-on-skin feel of caressing a shaved pubic area. That silky bare skin is heaven to inquiring fingers. Two shaved vulvas can make frottage delightfully intense.

Genital shaving is not to everyone's tastes—you might cringe at the thought of a razor coming anywhere near your tender parts, and the sight of bare genitals on an adult woman may be unappealing or even disturbing. You might find the increase in sensitivity not worth the itchiness as the hair grows in.

But those who shave their pubic areas swear by it. They wouldn't dream of giving up the pure eroticism of gently and carefully manipulating a razor (even an electric model) along the contours of such sensitive flesh.

You can shave yourself, of course, but being shaved by a partner is a special treat not to be missed. Having your outer labia and mons handled so delicately and slowly by a partner is very intimate. It certainly requires trust. As your partner painstakingly wields the razor, you can completely relinquish control and enjoy her entire attention to your needs. You can sink into a delicious reverie as you feel the indirect brush of a hand on your clitoris, the pinch of her fingers as she pulls your labia taut. By the time she's done, you may find that you're extremely turned on—your own juices may have lubricated the razor as much as her shaving gel! By all means, invite her to sample her handiwork.

How-to's of Genital Shaving

Start with a hot bath to soften your skin and your pubic hair. Wash thoroughly. Trim the hair as closely as possible with cuticle or other small sharp scissors. Pull the hair away from the skin to prevent nicking yourself with the scissors. Don't use clippers without a safety guard (even a #1 guard) because bare clippers can abrade the very delicate skin of your pubic area.

One trick to avoid irritation and nubs is to rub baby oil into your skin, let it dry for a few moments, and then lather up with shaving cream or gel. While just about any shaving cream or gel will do, you may want to select an unscented or even a hypoallergenic gel for best results. Many women prefer a gel to a foaming cream—it's easier to see what you're doing! Never scrape your sensitive genital area with a dry razor.

Use a high-quality disposable razor—one with a pivoting head to get into nooks and crannies. If you're shaving for the first time, grab a new razor halfway through. Don't reuse the razor.

---

*I am always a bit titillated and
ashamed of my shaved pussy. My lover
adores it and strokes it like a cat.*

Find a comfortable spot—leaning against the edge of the tub, sitting on the bathroom floor with your legs propped up—and a hand mirror. You might want to sit on a towel and prop the hand mirror up against the side of the tub. Begin by shaving in the direction of the hair growth. You'll gain confidence in safely wielding the razor as you work the areas farthest from your tender bits. Pull the area taut so that you have smooth skin to work with. Shave *with* the grain first; lather up, grab a new blade, and then very slowly and gently shave against the direction of the hair for a smooth feel. Move on to the next area; you can always come back to catch the stray hairs you've missed. (Shaving the same spot over and over will irritate your skin.)

You can shave the labia and inner thighs all the way down to the perineum; you can shave around the anus for smooth ass play (particularly satiny for rimming). There will often be a few stray hairs on the inside of the outer labia—you can catch these very carefully if you stretch your outer lips to their most-open position.

You can shave your mons bare or sculpt your pubes into an attractive shape. You can fashion a perfectly symmetrical triangle of thick hair or you can shave all but a tuft right at the top of the vulva—a handle for your partner.

When you're finished shaving, hop in the shower and rinse the area with antibacterial soap, such as Hibiclens. Pat dry. Don't use talcum powder, which has been linked to cancer. Moisturize with an unscented, quality lotion. Let your skin absorb the lotion and dry completely before getting dressed. You may feel a bit itchy after a day or so as the hairs grow back—you can shave again or take that itch as a signal that it's time for some attention!

Toys for Clitoral Play

What's the most essential item for clitoral play? Lube, of course! Even if your own natural lubrication is generous, it doesn't hurt to stock your toy bag with a supply of water-based or silicone lube. A wet clitoris will enjoy sensation far more than a dry one, and the perception of wetness will encourage your own lubrication as you become more aroused. Latex gloves, thoroughly coated with lube, will provide a very slippery surface for clitoral play.

Safer Clitoral Play

- Get a manicure. Make sure your nails are smoothly filed.

- Slip a glove or unlubed condom over the head of a Magic Wand or other vibrator with a tennis-ball style head. Always use a fresh condom or glove when switching sexual activities or partners.

- Use latex, nitrile, or vinyl gloves.

- Put on a fresh glove when you switch activities or partners.

- Don't share vibrators and other sex toys without cleaning in between uses.

- Use water-based or silicone lube. Don't use oil-based lube for clitoral stimulation.

- Don't allow bacteria from the anus to enter the vagina.

Silicone lubes, like ID Millennium and Eros, are far silkier than water-based lube. They're also latex-compatible and don't seem to ever dry up, which makes silicone lubes ideal for clitoral stimulation. (*Do not* use with silicone toys, as they will degrade the silicone in your dildo or butt plug.)

I need constant, unchanging stimulation, so a vibrator is best for me. I like indirect touching, not too hard, but fast and consistent.

Vibrators are the most popular toy for clitoral play. If your partner prefers intense direct clitoral stimulation, you may find that the consistent intensity of a vibrator works best for her. You can hold the vibrator, or she can—which will free up your hands for other pleasures. You can stroke her labia and the opening to her vagina, or hold the body of her clitoris gently between thumb and forefinger. See Chapter 15, "Sex Toys and Accoutrements."

As with vibrators, water spray from hand-held shower heads or Jacuzzi jets can provide intense stimulation. You can vary the water pressure by putting a finger over the hose or jet. Be careful *not* to spray water directly into the vagina, however.

Many women enjoy using nipple clamps for genital play. Clamps can be attached to the inner or outer labia. Like nipple clamps, labia clamps produce an intense sensation when they go on—and an even more intense sensation when they come off. If your partner is standing, you can try hanging one-ounce weights from the clamps for added sensation.

Clitoral Play—Safely

While hand-to-vulva contact is considered low risk for transmission of HIV and other STDs, consider using latex gloves. Blood or vaginal secretions coming in contact with small cuts or raw cuticles can increase your risk. (Pour vinegar over your hands. If you have any tiny cuts or open sores, you'll know!)

Herpes, HPV, and bacterial vaginosis can be transmitted via skin-to-skin contact. If you touch your partner's genitals and then touch your own, you can transmit bacteria or a virus. You need not have visible lesions or warts to transmit herpes or HPV; and you need not have visible breaks in the skin to acquire it. You can also transmit bacteria from the anus to the vagina; so change gloves or thoroughly wash your hands when changing activities.

Even with frottage—considered by most a safe activity—there's a slight risk of transmission of herpes or HPV with direct vulva-to-vulva contact.

See Chapter 16, "Safer Sex and Gynecological Health," for more information.

Where to Learn More

Want to become an expert at clitoral play? You can attend a Body Electric workshop or rent an instructional video, such as Annie Sprinkle and Joseph Kramer's "Fire in the Valley," which offers step-by-step instructions in female genital massage. See the "Resources" for more suggestions.

Suggested Web Links:

ANNIE SPRINKLE HOME PAGE
    www.heck.com/annie
BODY ELECTRIC
    www.bodyelectric.org/womens_index.htm

SOURCE OF QUOTE
Pat Califia, *Sex Magic: A Guide for Adventurous Couples* (Masquerade Books, 1993).

chapter nine

Oral Sex

*I love the feeling of my tongue
running over a hard clit.*

THERE'S NOTHING LIKE TONGUE AND LIPS ON VULVA—the taste, smell, and wet hot feel of a woman's engorged genitals. Many lesbians and bisexual women love to feel a partner's insistent tongue and lips sucking on their labia and erect clit.

Oral sex includes licking, biting, sucking, kissing, and flicking the clit, labia, and perineum, and penetration of the vagina and anus with the tongue. Mouth-to-vulva contact is called *cunnilingus*, *going down*, *muff diving*, *eating pussy*, *carpet munching*, or *tipping the velvet*. Mouth-to-anus sex is called *analingus* or *rimming*.

And while you won't find this sexual activity listed on the contents page of almost any other sex guide, many women love fellatio (also called *cocksucking*)—with a strap-on dildo attached to the body of a lesbian, bi woman, or female-to-male transsexual.

Oral sex, of course, is taboo in many Western cultures. We are taught to feel "dirty" down there. In parts of the United States, oral sex is still a crime. Yet some surveys report that oral sex is the favorite sexual activity of a significant number of people—both men and women. Certainly among lesbians, oral sex is extremely popular.

In 1999, the British lesbian monthly *Diva* published the results of a survey of 400 women readers of the magazine: 47 percent named oral sex as their favorite way to turn on a partner, and 38 percent rated cunnilingus as the form of "sexual attention they most liked to receive from a partner."[1] (An interesting discrepancy!)

> *I'm bisexual. I've had both female and male lovers tell me that they weren't into oral sex, which is my cue to tell them to get out of my bed!*

Cunnilingus

> *She sends shivers down my spine when she barely traces her tongue over me. The anticipation is enough to drive me crazy.*

Many lesbians and bisexual women are connoisseurs of the clitoris. What do we like about cunnilingus? The tongue and lips offer a delicious range of sensations that fingers simply can't match. There's nothing quite like that wet-on-wet combination of textures.

> *I love everything about giving oral sex. The smell, the taste, the way her lips and clit grow as I work them. The way she reacts when I slow down or speed up or suck her clit directly. The way she moans when I make my tongue hard and stick it in her cunt or lick her asshole.*

For some women, oral sex produces the most intense, toe-curling orgasms. And women whose clits are especially sensitive may respond to the subtleties of a tongue more readily than a hand or vibrator.

> *I love that my girlfriend comes so easily when I go down on her. Sometimes I lie on top of my vibrator while I go down on her, and that's very sexy for me.*

There's an intimacy in having someone's face so near to your genitals and in getting such a close-up on someone else's arousal. Having your most tender bits inside the mouth of your partner can make you feel vulnerable. You get to give up control. That sense of surrender may be quite freeing for you—and pure ecstasy for your partner.

I like knowing that I'm in complete control of her pleasure. I love feeling her melt in my mouth.

However, many women feel anything but submissive while furiously riding their lover's face!

It's just that sense of intimacy that can make cunnilingus such a powerful experience, one that for many requires a degree of trust. Having your partner's face between your legs can challenge your body image and self-acceptance. Do you really feel comfortable in your body? Do you feel beautiful opening up your sex for your partner's inspection?

My first girlfriend wouldn't go down on me, and we never talked about it. She wouldn't let me go down on her, either. I developed fear and shame that took several years to overcome. Now I love the taste of vaginal juice. I get wet imaging a cunt in my mouth. The softness, the sweetness, the wetness, and the intimacy of it completely turns me on. I think being comfortable with body fluids and being comfortable with intimacy helped me open up to enjoying oral sex.

Many women worry that they may smell or taste bad. Of course, jokes about women's genitals smelling like fish don't help matters. If you're concerned about how you will smell and taste, take a bath before sex. Next time you masturbate, taste your own juices. You may be surprised by how sweet you taste when you're turned on.

My lover has the most amazing lips. They are slightly swollen, and a beautiful walnut color, and always soft and warm.... And her thighs feel splendid next to my ears.

Going Down on Your Girl

Oral sex begins with talking. Women are as individual in their cunnilingus preferences as in any other aspect of sex. Don't assume your partner likes long languid licks, responds best to rapid flicks of the tongue, or wants you to bury your whole face in her fur. Ask her what she likes. You can even suggest that she take your head in her hands and put you exactly where she wants you. Play show-and-tell: show her—with your mouth on her vulva—how *you* like to receive oral sex and invite her to do the same for you. Demonstrate on *her* clit. Don't forget to tell her exactly what sends you over the edge.

Hair

I like bush. Furry girls. Getting pubes caught in your teeth—the whole enchilada.

Some women love the texture of pubic hair and the after-sex ritual of picking hairs from between their teeth. One woman wrote, "All of my best have been redheads. That's called 'going down in flames.' "

Others find those errant hairs a distraction. Hold her pubic hair aside with your hands—you can grip her hair between thumb and forefinger, hold her lips open, and even pleasure her with little tugs. You can give your partner a trim, shaving the outer labia and mons and trimming the outer pubic area in preparation for sex. Think of her coif as very creative foreplay. See shaving instructions in Chapter 8, "Clitoral Play," for details.

Blood

I absolutely loved the way her cunt tasted, with just a hint of iron.

The popularity of lesbian vampire erotica attests to the hold of blood on our imaginations. Are you a vampire? Some women love to taste a partner's menstrual blood during oral sex. In fact, some lesbians like to play vampire so much they seek out menstruating partners.

Others find blood contact unappealing—and even terrifying, given the fact that HIV, hepatitis, and other STDs can be transmitted through direct blood contact.

Some women have found safe ways to play with blood. The tangy, iron smell of your partner's blood can be an adequate substitute for taste—you can enjoy the aroma before covering her up with Saran wrap. You can don a glove and anoint her thighs and breasts with her own blood. She may even enjoy licking your gloved hand clean. Of course, if you're fluid-bonded (having unprotected sex only with each other), you and your partner can make an informed decision regarding oral sex during menstruation. See Chapter 16, "Safer Sex and Gynecological Health," for more information.

How-to's of Cunnilingus

- Be a tease. Start with indirect stimulation to warm her up.
- Lick and nibble her inner thighs, belly, and outer labia.
- Rub your entire face over her vulva.
- Nibble her inner labia; take each one into your mouth and suck.
- Put a drop of water-based lube on the genital side of a dental dam. As you tongue her clitoris, let the latex slide with your strokes. (Mark one side of the dental dam with a pen, so that when things get slippery, you know which side is which.)
- Circle her clit with the tip of your tongue. Experiment with different pressures and speeds.
- Stretch a piece of plastic wrap between her legs and around her waist like a loincloth—and then take a long lick from clit to butt.
- Penetrate her vagina with your tongue. Lick the area right below her urethra and just inside her vagina.
- Hum! Sound produces vibration. Your partner will feel as well as hear you groan as you pleasure her.
- Blow warm air over her vulva (*do not* blow directly into the vagina to avoid causing an air embolism).
- Flick your tongue rapidly over the glans, hood, and shaft of her clit.
- Flatten your tongue and rub it over her glans and shaft.
- Some women love the excruciating sensation of sharp nibbles on their tender parts. Some don't, so ask.

- Grab a glove—or two—and combine cunnilingus with penetration (vaginal or anal, or both). You can match the rhythms of your tongue with the thrusts of your fingers. Wrote one woman, "I love fingers inside of me while a tongue is licking me. When she uses the vibrator on me, too—whoa! Explosion!"
- If your partner likes G-spot stimulation (and you love the way she gushes when she comes), insert a finger or two and stroke her G-spot with that "come hither" gesture.
- You don't have to get her off by the clock. Back off, tease, go forward, tease some more. Stop and ask what feels best. Intensify your play as she gets more aroused.

Analingus

That musty scent along with her womanly scent is heaven.

You may never have thought that putting your mouth on your partner's anus would fill you with desire—or that having your partner's lips and tongue on yours would drive you wild. The idea of putting your mouth on someone's anus conjures responses ranging from memories of schoolyard insult ("Lick my ass!") to deep cultural taboo. But the delicacy and rich nerve endings of the anus combined with the soft, wet heat of tongue and lips provide for an extremely erotic array of sensations.

As with many turn-ons, there's no logic to what we love. One woman's ticket to ecstasy may be another's repulsion ("Rimming? Yuck! Why would anyone do that?").

Why would you want to tongue your partner's ass? Because she's so sensitive there, because rimming makes her squirm, and because the earthy taste and smell make you feel so primal—or simply because it's such a big taboo!

I'm not exactly sure why I love rimming a woman, but I do. I'm getting a bit wet just thinking about it.

What does having a tongue in your anus do for you? Well, the soft, subtle sensations can't be compared to anything else. Perhaps because the anus receives so little sexual attention, it's especially sensitive. The delicate, puckered mouth of your anus is ripe for play.

> *When my lovers rim me, they have me in the palm of their hand. I simply turn into flesh and bone offered up for their use.*

It's not uncommon to feel ambivalent about having a lover's tongue in your asshole. You may worry that you smell or taste bad, or that your lover will find feces there. While your concerns may be inhibiting, they may also be exciting—one woman wrote that rimming makes her feel like a "bad girl doing the forbidden," which is one reason she loves it!

> *I was so self-conscious that it wasn't entirely enjoyable. It felt good, though. If I could overcome my initial discomfort, I'm sure I'd love it.*

If you're concerned about cleanliness, you can shower, use dental dams or other barriers, or even have an enema before sex. There are usually small traces of fecal matter in the anus and rectum, and you can transmit hepatitis A, bacteria, or parasites through unprotected anal–oral contact. Licking her clitoris after rimming can lead to vaginal infections because bacteria from the anus may be carried by your tongue into her vagina.

Some women enjoy shaving the area around the anus—shaving makes for a smoother, cleaner feeling surface and as preparation for sex it can be a turn-on.

How-to's of Analingus
- Gently nibble the inner thighs and buttocks.
- Tickle the hairs around the anus with the tip of your tongue.
- Grab a glove and some water-based lube, to combine rimming with vaginal penetration or clitoral stimulation.
- Lightly circle her anus with your tongue.
- Flick your tongue rapidly against her opening.
- Lay your soft tongue flat against her anus and rub against the opening.
- Lick up and down her butt crack.
- Press your tongue into her opening.

Positions for Oral Sex

What are the best positions for oral sex? The ones that work for you, of course! You can lie between your partner's legs, especially if you like to maintain eye contact. This position has the added advantage of drawing on your upper body strength: prop yourself up on your elbows as you cup her ass cheeks in your hands, and then rock your upper body as you lick her clitoris.

But that's only the beginning. She may like to be licked while on her hands and knees. You can then slide your face under her—in either direction. You can lie on your back and have your partner straddle your face—it helps if she can steady herself by leaning on the wall or headboard.

Rear-entry is perhaps the easiest position for rimming because it affords good access to the anus. But most cunnilingus positions can be adapted for analingus as well.

You can bend over her vulva while kneeling at her side. With her legs spread wide and her hips raised, you can reach her anus as well. She can sit on the edge of her chair with you eagerly kneeling at her feet. She can stand over you.

With your partner on her knees or standing, her clit and labia hang down and can be sucked into your mouth; with your partner on her back with legs spread, her genitals are stretched out, providing a wider surface for your tongue.

Many women love the mutual stimulation of a "69" position, either lying on top of each other or side by side. You may find it difficult to concentrate on licking your partner when your brain has slipped down between your legs! Take turns pleasuring each other—there's no rule that performing 69 means you have to reach orgasm simultaneously.

And mutual pleasuring doesn't mean you both must like the same kinds of stimulation. You can penetrate your partner with fingers, a vibrator, or even your whole hand as her tongue and lips go to work on you. You can lick your partner while lying on a vibrator. Or you can simply reserve one hand for yourself!

What a Pain in the Neck!

A long session of oral sex can leave your neck feeling stiff or sore. You may have become so distracted that you may not have noticed the awkward position of your neck.

When my partner takes a very long time to come, my neck hurts!

There's no reason you should have to pay for your pleasure with a trip to the chiropractor. Choose a position that supports your neck. For instance, you can lie on your back with a pillow under your neck as your partner straddles your face. Or slip pillows under your partner's butt (or belly, if she's lying on her stomach) to prop her up.

If you're prone to neck and back pain, here's an opportunity to vary your repertoire. Combine oral sex with other forms of stimulation, make sure your partner is extremely aroused before you begin oral sex, or treat oral sex as a tasty appetizer—plug in the vibrator when it comes to the main course.

> *I thought I was going to have lockjaw once. She was lying back enjoying it, and I was thinking, "I love you, but come, for God's sake, or my tongue's going to commit suicide!"*

(Detachable) Cocksucking

> *The first time my girlfriend gave me a blow job, I came so hard I thought I'd shoot across the room.*

Many women love to give head to a gorgeous dyke with an eager cock. And many of those who "pack"—tucking a strap-on dildo into Levi's 501s or under a skirt—enjoy the attention of a blow-job.

So why would anyone want to suck a hunk of silicone? The allure of this practice is part fantasy and part sensation. Most women who enjoy woman-to-woman fellatio get off on the gender twist.

> *I love sucking lesbian cock. I'm really into the butch-on-butch thing.*

Getting on your knees before your partner is a bold admission of desire. Whether or not you associate cocksucking with submission, you can't miss the courage behind such a statement. You can feel your partner jump as you push the base of the dildo into her vulva. You can look up and watch her face as you lick the head of the dildo and slide it into your mouth. You're up close and personal with the very part of her that will drive you wild when she penetrates you vaginally or anally.

For the lucky one receiving that blow job? It's humbling to see your partner get on her knees for you. Having your partner worship your cock makes your gender fantasies come to life.

There's heat in holding her head and watching her take you inside her mouth. The pressure of her mouth and hands pushing the base of the dildo against your mons and clitoris may be enough stimulation to make you come. Many dildo-loving dykes name fellatio as their favorite way to reach orgasm.

I really can't explain the rush I get from a woman sucking my cock. It's almost like it's a real extension of me; and at times it has gotten me off!

You can combine silicone cocksucking with other kinds of stimulation. Your partner can lick her way to your butt or insert a finger into your anus or vagina. You can wear a butt plug and nipple clamps while your partner gives you head. You can slip a small battery-operated vibrator under the harness to provide direct clitoral stimulation or hold a wand-style vibrator between your thighs.

Sometimes while I'm getting sucked off, I'll put a pocket rocket on my clit and visualize myself shooting down her throat.

Some women combine fellatio with vaginal penetration. Vixen, the San Francisco–based toy company, makes a double-headed dildo angled just right for cocksucking. You can insert one end of the double-headed dildo into your vagina and offer up the other to be sucked. (See Chapter 15, "Sex Toys and Accoutrements.")

Vaginal penetration and cocksucking can be a confusing mix. Some women who enjoy fellatio with dildos don't want attention paid to their vagina. Then

Having my cock sucked changed my whole consciousness about gender and power.

again, she may like your fingers inside her vagina as you lean over to lick the tip of her dildo! Ask your partner what *she* likes.

How to Suck (Detachable) Cock

- Lick and nibble your partner's thighs and belly. Show her what a tease you can be!
- Slip an unlubed condom into your mouth. Roll it onto your partner's dildo.
- Hold the base of her dildo in your hand; this will help you control her thrusts into your mouth.
- Push the base of the dildo into her mons and clitoris.
- Circle the head of the dildo with your tongue.
- Grab a glove and slip your fingers behind the harness. You can stroke her clit as you suck the head of her cock.
- You can slide two fingers insider her vagina and stimulate her G-spot in rhythm to the thrusts of the dildo in your mouth.
- Keep a dental dam handy—while you're nibbling at her balls (featured on realistic models) or at the base of her dildo, you can lick your way to her vulva or anus.
- Alternate sucking on the tip of the dildo with slowly sliding the dildo into your mouth, taking more in each time.
- You can learn to relax your throat so that you can take more of her without gagging. You can practice in advance on your own dildo—or rent a how-to video, such as Nina Hartley's "Advanced Guide to Oral Sex."

Oral Sex—Safely

Even if you don't believe that women can transmit HIV via oral sex—and there simply haven't been enough studies to date to know for sure—we do know that other STDs *can* be transmitted through cunnilingus and analingus.

While the risk for transmitting HIV through unprotected cunnilingus (when no blood is present) is considered low, oral sex can transmit herpes and HPV (a virus linked to cervical cancer). Remember that if you like rough sex, with lots of biting, you may come in contact with blood even if your partner isn't menstruating.

When blood is present, the risk increases to include not only herpes and HPV, but also possible transmission of HIV, hepatitis C, and hepatitis B.

Analingus can transmit hepatitis A, anal herpes, anal warts, parasites, and possibly HIV. Many health advocates strongly recommend that you get a hepatitis A vaccine if you engage in unprotected rimming.

> *I contracted genital herpes from a girlfriend. I didn't know about safer sex. I was young, in love, and invincible. None of these things protected me. My girlfriend's pleasuring me orally was all it took. It is still a very sad thing for me. I do a lot of HIV/STD work. The ignorance among other young people is very scary. Lots of lesbians don't even know what a dental dam is.*

Of all of these STD risks, the most common story is that women routinely transmit herpes, HPV, and bacterial infections to each other through cunnilingus. Given the prevalence of these STDs, you'd think we'd all be stocking up o n Saran wrap and dental dams. But while many lesbians and bisexual women use latex barriers for oral sex, many do not. When lesbians let safer sex practices lapse, odds are they're going down.

> *Mmmmmmm, I love rimming. I don't take any precautions, and I know that I should. This is the one risky behavior I won't forego.*

So What's a Girl to Do?

> *The whole dental dam thing is a drag—if I can't go "down" naturally…then I don't bother.*

For some, STD risks are reason enough to opt out of oral sex. They don't want to risk transmitting or getting herpes and other STDs, but the thought of licking latex is unappealing.

Oral sex is not part of my sex life at all. My current partner will not engage in it with me due to the risks (I have had herpes since I first had sex!) and doesn't like dams or plastic wrap. In my professional life, I insist on dams or plastic wrap, and so most people decline!

Many women think barriers for oral sex will be awful, without even trying them. Gather some supplies (and your favorite sex partner!) and give them a whirl in the spirit of experimentation. You may surprise yourself.

Dental dams were designed to be used by dentists, of course, to keep your tongue and saliva out of the way while working on your teeth. The small squares of latex are thought to be effective barriers in preventing transmission of STDs during oral sex.

Since dental dams have a certain medical aesthetic—they are unattractive and a bit thick—sex-toy entrepreneurs came up with alternatives designed specifically for sex. One of these is the Glyde Lollyes dam—a sheer, 10" x 6" sheet of vanilla-scented latex, designed for sex—not root canals! Glyde dams are lightly powdered with cornstarch (which can be rinsed off before use). These are more expensive, but also more appealing than actual dental dams. Lixx also makes flavored dams for cunnilingus.

You can use plastic wrap—cheap and readily available. You can pull off as large a piece as you like and even wrap it around your partner like a loincloth. With plastic wrap, you can take a long forbidden lick from clit to vagina to butt and back again—without the worry of carrying bacteria from anus to vagina.

You can also cut up a latex glove or condom to use as a barrier (see illustration, Chapter 4, "The Road to Heaven Leads to You").

You may find rimming a more appealing practice when using a barrier. Try slipping an unlubed condom into your mouth, roll it over your tongue, and

Latex sorta tickles in a good way. Almost teasing, but I love being teased.

Safer Oral Sex

- Use dental dams, Saran wrap, or a cut-up glove or condom as a protective barrier for cunnilingus and analingus.

- Put a dab of water-based lube on the genital side of the barrier.

- Mark your side of the dental dam with a pen—so that if the dam slips you'll know which side's which.

- Always use a new dam or other barrier when you switch from rimming to cunnilingus, to reduce the risk of infection from anal bacteria.

- If you're allergic to latex, use plastic wrap or cut up a vinyl or nitrile glove.

- Use unlubed condoms on your dildos— always use a fresh condom when switching sexual activities or partners.

- If you enjoy rimming, consider getting a hepatitis A vaccination.

- Don't allow bacteria from the anus to enter the vagina.

- After unprotected rimming, rinse with antibacterial mouthwash before licking your partner's clitoris.

penetrate your partner as deeply as you desire. (Be aware that this technique works only if you keep your lips away from her exposed membranes.)

I'd never do rimming without a dental dam—I've known too many gay men who've suffered the medical repercussions of unprotected rimming.

Using a barrier, you can enjoy cunnilingus during menstruation without fear of blood contact. You can have oral sex with someone whom you might not feel you know well enough to put tongue to bare membrane.

You can even play with latex as a sex toy, creating sensations that might not be possible with your naked tongue. You can create a latex suction bubble, snap the latex against her genitals, put a dab of water-based lube on her side of the dam, and slide the latex over her clit. If you find direct clitoral stimulation to be too intense, latex can help by slightly decreasing sensation.

One complaint is that holding the dental dam in place occupies hands that could be put to better use elsewhere. The latex square tends to roll up. Holding it taut may require more effort than you care to devote to the task. You can buy a dental dam holder or modify a garter belt. Just shorten the garters to hold the latex square tightly against your vulva. If you sew on an extra set of fasteners, you can make a fashion statement with your Glyde dam and sheer black hose. Use your imagination—safer sex can become a fashion opportunity.

Is there a loss of intimacy in using dental dams and plastic wrap? Yes, many women find that licking and sucking a partner through a barrier diminishes taste, smell, texture, and that feeling of being so close to another's body.

Sometimes using latex makes me feel like I am not close enough. Especially with oral sex, because it is the taste of a woman that I find so pleasurable and arousing.

On the other hand, there's nothing like bonding over your mutual commitment to making healthy decisions. Talking about your sex histories, experimenting with safer-sex accoutrements, and laughing at your awkwardness can be very intimate. And while you're exploring the lube-and-latex options, you may just discover your partner's hottest fantasy of tongues and lips and her most tender places.

Suggested Web Links:

GLYDE DAMS
  www.sheerglydedams.com
THE SAFER SEX PAGES
  www.safersex.org/women/lesbianss.html

NOTES
  1. "The Diva Sex Report," *Diva*, January 1999, 16-20.

chapter ten

Vaginal Penetration

After a number of vaginal orgasms, I get this wonderful feeling
that I can only describe as being thoroughly done.

PENETRATIVE SEX IS INTIMATE. With your fingers and hands, you can feel every pulse and contraction of your partner's arousal and orgasm. With your partner's hand or dildo inside of you, you can enjoy a connection that is both immediate and emotionally powerful.

Penetration may be your preferred mode of reaching orgasm—you may enjoy multiple orgasms or wave upon wave of extended orgasm through vaginal penetration. Some women say they experience orgasms from vaginal penetration as deeper—"more bass than treble," as one woman wrote. Many women come most reliably from vaginal penetration combined with clitoral stimulation—from fingers, a vibrator, or tongue. Even if you don't reach orgasm through penetrative sex, you may crave that feeling of being filled. If it's your goal to reach orgasm through penetration (as either the insertive or the receptive partner), there are specific techniques you can try. Read on!

Take a Tour

A quick review of sexual anatomy will show that the clitoris is a system of engorging tissue—your clit isn't just the externally visible glans, but rather a

10 Myths About Vaginal Penetration

1. *If you want to be penetrated, you're not really a lesbian.* As Susie Bright says, "fucking is no more heterosexual than kissing."[1] Penetrative sex stimulates the sensitive outer third of the vagina, including the G-spot, and provides a delicious source of indirect clitoral stimulation. That feeling of fullness is both emotionally satisfying and physically pleasurable. Contrary to myth, nerve endings have no identity politics!

2. *Hands and fingers are fine for foreplay, but if it ain't a dick, it ain't sex.* Behind this myth is the notion that pleasure we produce with our hands—whether "digital penetration," "hand jobs," or masturbation—doesn't "count." Hands are dexterous. Fingers bend. They can produce a limitless variety of touch and motion, and can reach the G-spot more easily than a penis.

3. *Dildos are imitations of the real thing.* No, that strap-on dildo *is* the real thing—it's a *real* lesbian cock! Dildos have their own characteristics that make them uniquely well suited for sexual

pleasure—even women who have sex with men at times prefer a dildo to a penis. You can pick dildos for size, shape, and texture, and you can own one for every mood. Dildos aim to please—they stay hard, long after either partner's orgasm. Dildos go back into the drawer after sex.

4. *I like penetration, but if I wanted something in me that looked like a penis, I'd go out and get a man.* You can find dildos to suit every taste (so to speak). Some are realistic, with veins, balls, and glans (you can even buy a dildo modeled after a famous porn star). Others are abstract, like Vixen's collection of variously shaped dildos that come in all colors and even swirl patterns. See Chapter 15, "Sex Toys and Accoutrements."

5. *But I can't come from penetrating my partner.* For some strap-on studs, getting off isn't the point. But if you'd like to reach orgasm while penetrating your partner, see below.

"pyramid-shaped mass of erectile tissue."[2] Clitoral tissue cradles the urethra, and the crura extend back to the vaginal walls. During penetration, the clitoris is stimulated indirectly through the walls of the vagina.

Most women find the area of the vagina nearest the opening to be the most responsive to touch, which makes sense since the outer third of the vagina contains the most nerve endings. The G-spot is located on the front wall of the vagina, fairly close to the opening.

6. *Women who strap on dildos want to be men.* Strap-on studs may identify as transgendered—some as butch lesbians and some as FTMs. And some butches and FTMs like to get penetrated! Some women wear strap-ons with garters, sheer fishnet stockings, and heels. You don't have to associate strap-on play with gender at all—you can wear a dildo to penetrate your partner just because you like how it feels.

7. *Fisting is dangerous.* Not if you do it right. See "Vaginal Fisting," below.

8. *If you get fisted, you'll end up all stretched out (and you won't be satisfied with a mere finger, dildo, or penis).* The muscles at the opening of the vagina get stronger with use, not weaker. If you're concerned about maintaining muscle tone, do your PC exercises. (See Chapter 3, "Anatomy and Sexual Response.") Will you be spoiled by the intensity of that fist inside you? Yes!

9. *If you like to get fucked, you're a "bottom."* Vaginal penetration can be part of a dominance/submission scene, with the top fisting her submissive partner or penetrating her with a strap-on or hand-held dildo. Conversely, the top can be the receptive partner, directing her partner's actions with great menace and authority. ("Get that cock in me! Now!") The bottom can feel very compliant on her knees between her top's legs. Of course, many women who enjoy penetrative sex have no interest in power play whatsoever. Penetration simply feels good. See Chapter 13, "Play Nice! (...or Else)."

10. *Women who crave penetration are really bisexual (or even heterosexual).* Maybe, maybe not. One woman wrote, "I never enjoyed vaginal penetration until I identified as a lesbian." The hidden fear behind this myth is that your partner will reject you for a man. Many lesbians who have no interest in men love vaginal penetration, as do many bisexual women. Regardless of whether your partner enjoys sex with men, at this moment it is *your* hard cock, poised expectantly between her legs, that she desires. Enjoy!

Take a tour of your own vagina before inviting a partner in. When you reach inside with your fingers pointing toward the front wall of your vagina, you can find your G-spot by stroking in a "come hither" motion. Some women find G-spot stimulation really pleasurable, and others find it irritating. Using your fingers or a firm, curved dildo, experiment with movement and pressure. You can locate your cervix and note how your uterus lifts and your vagina balloons out as you approach orgasm. It's much easier to tell a lover how to please you when you know what you like! See Chapter 3, "Anatomy and Sexual Response," and Chapter 5, "Masturbation."

Finger Fucking

Your fingers are extremely communicative. You can feel and transmit very subtle sensations with your fingers. Your fingers are also dexterous. They can bend and reach to explore every nook and cranny. You can use your fingers as a prelude to something, well, bigger—more fingers, a hand, or a dildo—or as the main attraction. Not every woman wants four fingers inside her vagina; and those who do may enjoy the feeling of slowly adding fingers one at a time.

You can caress the opening of the vagina, and your partner can squeeze your fingers as you find her most sensitive spots. You can easily reach her G-spot by angling your fingers toward the front wall of the vagina. Try caressing her G-spot with varying pressure and speed, as you would the glans and hood of her clit.

As the receptive partner, you can push out toward your partner's hand; your G-spot will be easily apparent as an area of tissue that's spongier and rougher than the rest of your vagina.

You can use one hand for penetration, reserving the other for clitoral stimulation. The finger circling her clit can match the rhythms of the finger thrusting inside her. You can hold a vibrator to her clit, or she can touch herself—leaving you to concentrate on her vagina. With two or three fingers you can rapidly thrust in and out, pumping at a pitch that you couldn't possibly sustain with a strap-on dildo.

Vaginal Fisting

When I'm being fisted, I am all cunt.

Fisting (also called *handballing* or *fist fucking*) is the practice of inserting a whole hand inside a woman's vagina (or anus—see Chapter 11, "Anal Penetration"). Contrary to its name, the balled-up fist isn't forced past the vaginal opening but is slowly and gently inserted. After the hand is inside, it's curled into a ball—hence the term *fisting*.

Fisting is about trust and desire. You have to *want* to be fisted to open so dramatically to another human being—and you have to trust your partner to allow her entry in such an intimate way. While not everyone can be fisted—and a particular hand may be too big for a particular vagina—fisting is more a matter of arousal than anatomy.

Those who love fisting speak of the primal connection of having one's entire hand inside the body of another human being. For emotional intimacy, nothing surpasses fisting, they say. You can feel every ripple and pulsation of your partner's arousal. Deep inside her body, it feels as if you have the core of her sexual power literally in the palm of your hand.

For women who crave deep penetration, fisting satisfies that need to be completely filled. You can ride every subtle movement of your partner's hand into an ocean of sensation. You can completely surrender to the overwhelming intensity of being inexorably penetrated.

How does fisting work? The vagina is quite elastic. After all, it stretches to accommodate a baby during birth. When you're sexually aroused, your whole vagina expands, opens, and balloons out. As you near orgasm, your vagina becomes quite spacious.

Some women discover fisting almost by accident: One particularly hungry day, when three or even four fingers aren't enough, your vagina engulfs your partner's hand. However, most women come to fisting more intentionally.

Fisting requires communication, patience, and lube—lots of lube. The receptive partner takes control to receive her partner's fist. She must communicate how much, how fast, how intensely those fingers, and finally that hand, can enter. To do so, she needs to be aware of her body. She needs to know what feels good and what doesn't, and what she needs and wants—and to be able to communicate these to her partner even when the sensations are overwhelming.

Unless you and your partner are veteran fisters, this is not an activity for a lunch-break quickie. Take your time. Before you even *think* about penetration, make sure the receptive partner is thoroughly turned on.

Snap on a latex glove and coat your entire hand with a water-based lube—front and back, up to the wrist. Begin with two fingers. Then three fingers. Then four. Tuck your thumb into the palm of your hand. Try to make your hand as skinny as possible—fisting how-to guides speak of folding your hand into the shape of a duck's bill. (See the "Bibliography.")

Enter her vagina up to the widest part of the hand, with your palm facing the front wall of her vagina and your knuckles facing her tailbone. At this point, move only by millimeters. Stop frequently to add more lube. Talk to your partner—ask her what feels good and what doesn't. Maintain eye contact. Breathe with her. You can place the palm of your free hand on her chest or hold her hand. Connect with her in any way that works for the two of you.

Some women love the circular pressure of a scooping motion on the fully stretched vaginal opening. You may be able to rotate your way inside of her. Or, you may be able to push straight in; you'll feel a "pop" and your hand will disappear.

But what if it hurts? Most likely, if you are four fingers deep and about to sink your entire hand into your partner, the pain comes from the widest part of your hand pushing against the ring of muscles at the opening of her vagina. The bones of your hand also may be pressing painfully against her pelvic bones.

Just as the vagina opens with arousal, it shuts down with fear or stress. Don't try to force your hand inside of her. Fisting is not supposed to hurt. Back off to

*The first time she put her hand inside
me, I was looking into her eyes;
it was very, very intimate. She says that
she can feel my orgasm start before I do; I love
letting her be that close to me.*

three fingers or even two. Add more lube. You might try to enter her from a different angle. Let her take the lead.

Some women open more easily after orgasm. If your partner is rocking up against your hand, squeezing her thighs, and contracting around your fingers—in other words, if she's working up to a colossal orgasm—you may want to ride that orgasm with her. After she comes, stay inside, moving very slowly. Let her arousal build back up again. You may find that her vagina opens wide enough for your hand to slip though.

Other women open to their fullest during a long session of penetrative sex *without* orgasm. The more turned on they get, the more their vagina opens. You can postpone your partner's orgasm, a sweet torture all its own. Slow her down. Still your fingers. Ask her to relax the muscles of her pelvis and thighs, and to breathe with you, slowly and deeply. For the woman who loves to wrap herself around a finger or dildo, this will seem counterintuitive—but it works!

That having been said, fisting isn't something you "make" happen. Don't be goal oriented. Both partners need to be relaxed and open to possibility.

What to do when you get your hand inside your partner? Ball up your hand into a fist. Immediately. And then be still as your partner adjusts to the overwhelming reality of your hand filling her vagina—not to mention her consciousness!

When your partner is ready, you can move your hand. Remember that a small movement to you is a tidal wave to her. Some women like a slow rotation from the wrist in very small, subtle, corkscrew movements. Others like a gentle thrusting movement—just a centimeter forward and back, slowly and then more rapidly as she gets turned on. Eventually she may become so open that you're able to thrust in and out, pulling your hand completely out of her vagina and working your hand inside her over and over. The intensity of this is indescribable.

Some women like the pressure on their cervix that comes with deep penetration. That doesn't mean banging on the cervix, which is delicate and can be bruised easily. Here's where you can appreciate the "ballooning" of the vagina just before orgasm. Depending on her menstrual cycle and the location of her cervix, you may be able slip your hand behind her cervix.

In fisting, your partner can ride the edge of her orgasm for a long, long time. In fact, some women like to be fisted endlessly with little thought of coming. Others will begin climbing to the peak of an extended orgasm the moment your fist begins to move. You can combine fisting with many other sources of stimulation, including vibrators, nipple clamps, and even a small butt plug. Some women like to use a vibrator on their clit while being fisting. Others prefer their own fingers.

Don't yank your hand out of your partner's vagina. Getting out is best handled as gently as going in. If your partner has clamped down on your hand, you may have to slowly work your way out.

Fisting can be a vulnerable experience for both partners. Allow time to cool down together.

Strap-on Dildos

Dildos are perhaps the world's oldest sex toys. You can hold a dildo in your hand or wear it in a harness, freeing up your hands for other pleasures.

Dildos come in all shapes and sizes. A dildo appropriate for strap-on sex has a flared base so that it will not slip out of the harness. Harnesses come in several different styles.

Single-strap (thong–style) harnesses feature a strap that goes between the legs. Some women love the stimulation of the center strap; others don't like a strap between their legs. You can attach a cuff to hold a dildo or butt plug in place on the center strap. Some women find these harnesses to be the most stable.

Two-strap (jock–style) harnesses have straps that go around the thighs and butt much like a jockstrap; they tend to position the dildo lower on your body, right over your mons. They may provide more stimulation for the wearer.

Thigh harnesses wrap around one thigh, with the dildo protruding out of a ring in the fabric. Some women find movement with the thigh harness easier and more natural. If you like to hump a partner's thigh, this harness may be for you!

You'll learn all about selecting dildos and harnesses in Chapter 15, "Sex Toys and Accoutrements."

Wielding a strap-on takes practice; you may feel very self-conscious the first time you look in the mirror and see a dildo bobbing between your legs. Try wearing the dildo and harness when you're alone. You can even masturbate while wearing your new strap-on.

Use your fingers to explore your partner's vagina before you penetrate her with a dildo. You can learn the size and shape of her vagina and discover what feels best to her. Roll a condom onto your dildo and apply plenty of water-based lube. Use your hand to guide the dildo into her. Go slowly and watch her face.

If you're the receptive partner, you're in charge during strap-on sex. Here's an opportunity to hone your communication skills. Since your partner has no nerve endings in the tip of her dildo (much as it may feel that she does at times), she can't know if she's painfully banging your cervix unless you tell her. Do you want your partner to grind slowly and deeply into you? Do you want her to thrust faster? Harder? Tell her!

The thrusting of the dildo inside you may provide enough indirect clitoral stimulation to bring you to orgasm. Just the fantasy of a woman with a hard cock may be enough to make you come. You can also combine vaginal penetration with direct clitoral stimulation. You can stimulate your clitoris with a vibrator or your fingers as your partner is penetrating you. Your partner can slip a vibrating cock ring onto her dildo; she can stimulate your clitoris as she grinds into you. In the rear-entry position, she can reach around and touch your clit as she penetrates you.

But what about the thrill of having your partner come with her dildo deep inside you? What about the insertive partner who wants to reach orgasm while penetrating her partner?

When she's doing me with a dildo
I feel wild and slutty—
it's just good rough dirty sex.

Fairy Butch's Stimulation Tips for Strap-On Sex

- Rub your clitoris against the center strap of a thong-style harness.

- Wrap a leather cuff around the center strap of a thong-style harness to hold a vibrating egg against your clitoris or a dildo inside your vagina—or both!

- Place a vibrating cock ring around the shaft of your dildo and tuck it behind your harness.

- Press the flange (base) of a vibrating dildo against your clitoris to magnify friction.

- Use a dildo with nubs molded into the back of the flange and position it to stimulate your clitoris.

- Use a butt plug for hands-free anal stimulation.

- Wear a Leather Butterfly pouch behind your harness to hold a vibrating egg to stimulate your clitoris.

- Use the pounding action of penetration to manipulate the crura of your clitoris as you thrust into your partner.

- Have your partner penetrate your vagina while you are wearing a jockstrap-style harness.

- Use two thigh harnesses to allow both partners to act as insertive and receptive partners simultaneously.

- Use a two-pronged dildo or vibrator to stimulate your vagina and anus simultaneously as you penetrate your partner.

Just the idea of thrusting your strap-on dildo into a partner's vagina may be enough to make you come. Perhaps the base of the dildo rubbing against your clitoris provides the stimulation you need. If you require direct clitoral stimulation to reach orgasm, you can strap a battery-operated vibrator, such as an egg vibe, over your clit. Your partner can hold a Magic Wand between your thighs. You can reach under your harness and touch yourself as you penetrate your partner. You can also wear a vibrating dildo or butt plug.

For some strap-on studs, getting off isn't the point. They like seeing the dildo penetrating a partner's vagina and giving a partner all that pleasure. In fact, for some women, that's the best thing about strap-on sex—an enthusiastic partner whose cock stays hard!

How-to's of Vaginal Penetration

- As the receptive partner, take the lead. Tell your partner exactly how you want to be penetrated.
- Roll a condom onto your partner's strap-on. Lube her up!
- As the insertive partner, make sure your partner is really turned on before you enter her.
- Use lube—lots of lube—even if she seems fairly wet to you. You can warm the lube by running hot water over the bottle before you begin to play.
- Snap on a latex glove—lubricated latex will make your fingers and hand ultra smooth.
- Even if your intention is to fill your partner with your entire hand or your strap-on dildo, start with one finger. Build up slowly.
- You can take your partner's wrist in hand and guide her inside you.
- Tease her—give her less than she wants, and then a little more.
- Bring out the toys—add nipple clamps, bondage, vibrators, and butt plugs to penetrative sex.
- You can lean over and lick her clitoris while pumping your fingers or a hand-held dildo in and out of her vagina.
- Use two hands—you can slip the fingers of one hand into your partner's vagina while the other hand attends to her anus. Your fingers can "meet" through the thin wall of tissue separating the vagina from the anus. (Do not allow bacteria from the anus to come in contact with the vagina.)
- You can rotate your hips or move them in a steady in-and-out motion to vary the thrusts of the dildo.
- Place the palm of one hand just above your partner's pelvis bone and press—you can feel your fingers thrusting against her G-spot.
- As the receptive partner, you can wrap your legs around your partner's hips and rock her dildo into you. You can use her harness to pull her into you more deeply or to control the pace of her thrusts.
- Experiment with two-handed fisting. Hold your hands with palms together, and slip one hand in as the other slides out, rubbing your palms together.
- Hold a vibrator against your partner's clitoris—or your own!

Positions for Vaginal Penetration

Kneeling or sitting between your partner's legs. With your partner lying on the bed, place yourself between her legs. This position is great for fisting, finger fucking, or penetration with a hand-held dildo.

You can maintain eye contact. You can reach your partner's breasts and belly—and she can reach yours! You can reach both vagina and anus. You can bend over and lick your partner's clitoris as you penetrate her.

There's plenty of room for her to hold a vibrator to her clitoris or to touch herself. By raising her legs, she can adjust the angle of entry. For deepest penetration, she can rest her ankles on your shoulders or bend her knees almost to her chest and hook her arms behind her calves.

Missionary. The missionary position may sound old-fashioned, but it's ideal for intimate strap-on sex. With your partner lying on her back, you lie between her legs. This position works well with the thigh harness as well as harnesses that strap around the hips.

You can enjoy long, deep kisses and up-close eye contact. You can grind your pelvises together. The receptive partner can wrap her arms and legs around your shoulders and hips. You can slip a vibrator between your bodies.

This position works well in a sling. Many lesbians sing the praises of the sling. A sling is a type of hanging chair that fully supports your weight, allowing all your muscles to relax. With no muscle tension, many women find they can better enjoy penetrative sex. Slings can be constructed from nylon webbing, canvass, leather or rubber. They generally hang from eyebolts in a ceiling or wall, or from a freestanding frame.

Receptive partner on top. Here's a strap-on position in which the receptive partner can most easily control the depth of penetration. The insertive partner can sit on a chair, lie on her back, or recline in a sling while you straddle her, raising and lowering yourself on the dildo. This is a good position if you can't bear weight on you.

Not only do you control depth, you can also control the speed and movement. You can thrust in slow circling motions or pump as hard and fast as you like. By squeezing your PC muscles around the dildo, you can grind the base of the dildo into your partner's pelvis.

In a chair or sling, you can wrap your arms around each other and enjoy the intimacy of face-to-face contact. With the insertive partner lying on her back, she can stroke your clit or hold a vibrator for you. This position works well with the thigh harness.

Rear entry. Rear entry is the position often associated with anal sex. It's also great for all kinds of vaginal penetration—finger fucking, fisting, and penetration with a hand-held or strap-on dildo. The receptive partner kneels on hands and knees, with the insertive partner kneeling or standing behind her. This is a good position if either partner can't bear weight on her.

> *The picture in my head of me bent over, getting fucked from behind, is where my orgasm comes from.*

Rear entry provides for the deepest penetration and most direct G-spot stimulation. This is a good position for those who desire intense, hard thrusting. The insertive partner can hold onto her partner's hips as she drives the dildo into her vagina. The receptive partner has freedom of movement—she can rock backward, slamming against her partner's dildo or hand.

The receptive partner can easily touch herself. She can also lower herself onto the bed and rub her vulva against the sheets or her hand.

Side by side. Like the missionary position, lying on a bed side by side is a very intimate way to enjoy penetrative sex. With the receptive partner's leg thrown over your hips, you can slip a dildo into her vagina as you wrap your arms around her, enjoying her kisses and face-to-face closeness. You can enjoy simultaneous finger fucking in this position. This is a great position for slow, sensuous strap-on sex. This is a good position if either partner can't bear weight on her. Side-by-side sex works well with the thigh harness, as well as harnesses that fit around the hips.

Standing. Many lesbians entertain the fantasy of pressing a partner up against a wall, lifting her skirt, and slipping fingers deep inside her—or a strap-on, or even a whole hand. Standing sex carries with it a sense of urgency—as if you can't wait long enough to find a bed.

Of course, size is a factor. You have to be well-matched to enjoy strap-on sex standing up—unless one of you is much taller than the other and can pick up her partner. You can make use of a staircase to equalize height, too. This position is useful if the receptive partner can't bear weight.

Toys for Vaginal Play

When it comes to toys for penetrative sex, lube tops the shopping list. Water-based lube is a *must* for pleasurable vaginal play—whether you plan to use dildos or your own fingers to penetrate your partner. Combined with gloves, water-based lube will turn your hand into a slick surface. (Use only water-based lubes in the vagina; oil-based lubes, such as Crisco, don't rinse out of the vagina easily and can lead to vaginal infections.)

Your basic eight-inch silicone strap-on is only the beginning when it comes to dildo play. The newest innovation in dildo design is Cyberskin, a remarkably realistic-feeling material.

If you wear a harness with a center strap, you can add a harness cuff to hold a dildo or butt plug—you can even slip a vibrating dildo or butt plug inside the harness cuff for added stimulation.

Safer Vaginal Penetration

- Get a manicure. Make sure your nails are smoothly filed.

- Use latex, nitrile, or vinyl gloves.

- Use water-based lube.

- Put on a fresh glove when you switch activities or partners.

- Don't share dildos and vibrators without cleaning in between uses.

- Use condoms on your dildos. Always use a fresh condom when switching sexual activities or partners.

- Don't allow bacteria from the anus to enter the vagina.

Some women like to play with double dildos—you can penetrate your partner *and* yourself simultaneously. Newer designs are angled for easy use. Some have flexible spines, allowing them to be bent to the precise angle that works for you.

Hand-held dildos are great for G-spot stimulation; some, such as the S-shaped Crystal Wand, are designed for just that purpose.

You can find a large variety of battery-operated vibrators designed for penetrative sex. See Chapter 15, "Sex Toys and Accoutrements," for more information.

Vaginal Penetration—Safely

While penetration with fingers, hands, and dildos is considered very low risk for transmission of HIV, unprotected penetrative sex can tranmit STDs such as herpes, HPV, and chlamydia from woman to woman.

Ungloved hands make finger fucking and fisting risky. Your fingernails can scratch the lining of your partner's vagina, providing a transmission route for bacteria and STDs. Ragged cuticles or small cuts on your hand can provide a transmission route for STDs that may be present in your partner's menstrual blood or vaginal secretions.

Shared dildos can lead to vaginal infections as well as transmission of some STDs. Use a condom and clean your dildos with antibacterial soap.

Herpes, HPV, and bacteria can be transmitted via skin-to-skin contact. If you touch your partner's genitals and then touch your own, you can transmit bacteria or a virus. You need not have visible lesions or warts to transmit herpes or HIV, and you need not have visible breaks in the skin to acquire it. You can also transmit bacteria from the anus to the vagina; change gloves or thoroughly wash your hands when changing activities.

Even if you're monogamous and don't use latex barriers with your partner, some safer-sex considerations still apply.

First, keep your hands clean. Not just lather-and-rinse clean, but seriously clean. Make sure there's no grime around the nails—if you choose not to wear gloves for sex, perhaps you should consider wearing them for work. Don't touch yourself and then your partner without washing your hands.

Second, get a manicure. Trim your nails as closely as possible, until there's no white showing. Make sure your cuticles are smooth. Remove hangnails. Does that mean that femmes with fabulous nails are prohibited entry? No way! Here are a few precautions: File the nails until smooth, making sure there are no jagged edges or sharp points. Before you slip on that latex glove, grab some cotton balls. Place bits of cotton padding over the sharp ends of your nails—then pull on the latex glove. Voilà! If you don't use gloves, you must be very conscious of the location of your nails. Make sure that only the pads of your fingers make contact with the vaginal walls. Fisting may be easier for you than finger fucking—you can tuck your nails into your palm.

Finally, don't forget to urinate before and after vaginal penetration. Emptying your bladder before penetrative sex will help make room for a dildo or your partner's hand. Peeing after sex can also help prevent urinary tract infections.

See Chapter 16, "Safer Sex and Gynecological Health," for more information.

Where to Learn More

You'll find workshops on strap-on sex, fisting, and other techniques at some sex boutiques. In San Francisco, Karlyn Lotney (aka Fairy Butch) offers classes that cover the basics of strap-on sex. In the Boston area, Grand Opening's Kim Airs has offered workshops on G-spot play and the "ins and outs" of lesbian sex. In Toronto, Good for Her has offered workshops on vaginal fisting.

If you can't find a workshop or class, you can view lesbians and bisexual women having penetrative sex by renting a lesbian sex video. The "San Francisco Lesbians" series features numerous scenes of strap-on sex. (See the "Resources.") You can also read online advice columns geared toward lesbians, such as Ask Aphrodite and Ask Fairy Butch.

Suggested Web Links:

ASK APHRODITE
    www.a-womans-touch.com
ASK DR. MYRTLE
    www.a-womans-touch.com
ASK FAIRY BUTCH
    www.fairybutch.com

NOTES
1. Susie Bright, *Susie Sexpert's Lesbian Sex World* (Cleis Press, 1990, 1998), 15.
2. Susan Williamson, reporting O'Connell's findings in *Today's Life Science*. See also Helen E. O'Connell, et al., "Anatomical Relationship Between Urethra and Clitoris," *Journal of Urology*, vol. 159, 1892–97, June 1999.

SOURCE OF SIDEBAR
"Fairy Butch's Stimulation Tips for Strap-On Sex" is adapted from *The Ultimate Guide to Strap-On Sex* by Karlyn Lotney (Cleis Press, 1999).

chapter eleven

Anal Penetration

*Anal penetration is very intimate sex play for me.
I love the whole process of building trust, and the slowness of it.*

ANAL SEX IS DELICIOUS. The delicate folds of the anus and the tender lining of the rectum are rich in nerve endings and transmit very subtle sensations. Even a slender fingertip can produce enormous anal pleasure.

Many women say they experience their most intense orgasms through anal penetration, especially when combined with clitoral stimulation. Perhaps you like anal penetration because you experience indirect G-spot stimulation through pressure on the walls of the rectum. You may relish the naughty thrill of engaging in a form of sexuality that's so taboo.

The keys to pleasurable anal sex are communication, relaxation, and lubrication. The women of Toys in Babeland in New York and Seattle call these their butt-play mantra: "You can never have too much of any of those three, so talk about it, breathe deep, slap on more lube than you think is necessary, start slow, and have fun!" [1]

Take a Tour

Make yourself comfortable—take a hot bath, put on some relaxing music, light some candles, and unplug the phone. Grab a hand mirror and your favorite lube.

Slip on a latex glove. (If you'd rather not use a glove, make sure your nails are smoothly filed and your hands clean and soft. See "Basic Preparation.")

You can sit on the bed or lean back in a plush chair. Hold the mirror in between your legs; or, for an even better view, kneel or squat over the mirror. Viewing the puckered folds of the anus, you can appreciate how delicate it is. We're often so crass in how we refer to our asses that we forget how tender we are there.

Rub a lubed finger over the opening. Get used to the feeling of your anus being stimulated. Slip just the tip of your lubed finger inside. Notice the heat you generate, the firm grip of your sphincter muscles on your finger, and the pulsing sensation as the anus becomes aroused and the tissues engorge with blood.

You have two muscles at the opening of your anus: the external and internal sphincters. The external sphincters are voluntary muscles—you can flex the external sphincter as you squeeze your PC muscles. The internal sphincters are involuntary—they react automatically to stimuli like pleasure or fear. However, like other involuntary muscles, they can be trained.

If you poke directly at the anus, the sphincter muscles will clamp down in an automatic response much like the blinking of an eye. This response, which some sex educators call the "anal wink," [2] explains many bad anal sex experiences. Someone attempts to enter you by poking a finger or toy into your anus. Your internal sphincter closes against the intrusion. It hurts. You tell the errant partner to remove the finger, butt plug, or dildo. Next time a finger, dildo, or butt plug nears your anus, your unforgiving sphincter clamps down against the memory of that painful intrusion.

Rather than conditioning your anus for pain, you can condition it for sexual enjoyment. With relaxation, communication, and lots of lube, you can teach your sphincters to anticipate pleasure.

The anus opens into the anal canal, which is only an inch or two long. If you reach a lubed finger a bit deeper inside your anus, you can feel the tight anal canal opening into the roomier rectum. The rectum is four to six inches long and curves in a gentle S shape. The rectum ends in the rectosigmoidal junction (the top of the S), which leads to the colon. When you feel the need to defecate, you are feeling feces pressing on the rectosigmoidal junction. (Unlike the vagina,

10 Reasons to Have Anal Sex

1. Anal penetration feels fabulous!

2. Relaxation. Many of us hold tension in the anal area. Anal penetration provides a great way to get a massage—from the inside.

3. Anal penetration can help heal and even prevent hemorrhoids.[3]

4. You can make friends with a part of your body you've been taught (at best) to ignore.

5. You can have it all. On your knees, with your partner penetrating you anally from behind, you can press a vibrator to your clit, reach your fingers inside your vagina, stimulate your G-spot, and even feel your partner's fingers, dildo, or hand through the thin wall of tissue separating your vagina from your rectum.

6. Anal penetration can provide indirect G-spot and clitoral stimulation.

7. You can have mind-blowing orgasms.

8. Because anal penetration is associated so strongly with stereotypes about gender and power, it's great for playing out many fantasies. You can be a submissive girl being taken by her dominant lover. With dildos and harnesses, you can pretend you're gay boys in the backroom of a bar.

9. You can feel terribly naughty! Nothing like breaking a taboo to make you feel deliciously bold.

10. Anal penetration can create a sense of vulnerability and surrender. You can feel utterly taken. You can give it up in a big way.

---

there's no "end" to your rectum; objects really *can* get lost in there. See the guidelines later in this chapter for selecting anal toys.) The lower portion of the rectum curves toward the front of your body; the upper portion curves back toward your spine. Your fingers are probably not long enough to follow these curves, but you can use a slender dildo to find the point at which your rectum curves forward. Of course, each person's anus and rectum are unique.

Like the clitoris, the tissue of the anus and rectum engorge with blood as you become aroused. Your mirror may reveal your anus opening as you get turned on. The rectum also expands—not as readily as your vagina, of course, but you can fit a finger, a dildo or penis, a butt plug, or even an entire hand inside your butt. Unlike the vagina, the rectum does not produce its own lubrication.

The lining of the anus and rectum is very delicate and will tear easily—reasons to be extremely careful in choosing insertive anal toys and to tend to your manicure.

In biological males, the prostate gland, which is located on the front wall of the rectum, several inches in from the opening, can respond to stimulation similarly to the G-spot. If you play with a male-to-female transsexual (MTF), remember that she *has* a prostate gland. Ask her whether or not she finds prostate stimulation pleasurable.

Basic Preparation

> *I like giving myself an enema with a red rubber bottle and hose, but it must be private. I love the way it feels when the warm water goes inside me.*

Here are some suggestions for preparing for anal penetration:
- *Get a manicure.* Even if your ultimate goal is to penetrate your partner with a dildo, you'll most likely start with your hands. Trim your nails as closely as possible. File your nails until they feel smooth against the skin of your face. Remove hangnails. Use lotion to soften your cuticles. (If you want to keep your nails long, slip cotton balls over your nails before you put on a glove.)
- *Wear a glove.* Even if you and your partner are fluid-bonded, wearing a glove will enhance anal sex. Why? The glove will protect your partner from your nails and will provide a super-smooth surface.
- *Eat sensibly.* Make sure your diet includes plenty of fiber and whole foods. Avoid sesame seeds and strawberries—or any foods containing nuts or small seeds, which will scrape rectal tissue.
- *Empty your bowels* before you play.
- *Bathe.* Soaking in a hot tub will relax you as well as render you deliciously clean and pink.
- *Give yourself an enema.* Give yourself an enema. Some people prefer to have an enema before anal penetration. Fisting experts recommend enemas before deep anal play. You'll find detailed information on enemas in Tristan Taormino's *The Ultimate Guide to Anal Sex for Women.* Here are some enema basics: You can find enema kits, bulb syringes, and enema bags in any pharmacy, and nozzles that attach to your shower head in mail-order catalogs (see "Resources"). For

the novice, the simplest enema solution will be to purchase a commercial-prepared enema kit, such as Fleet, empty out the solution and rinse well. Commercial enema preparations contain laxatives and harsh chemicals that can irritate your rectum. Plain, filtered water heated to 100° F is the best choice. Gently squeeze the warm water into your rectum until you feel full. Wait a few minutes and evacuate the water and any feces in your bowels. Repeat until the water you expel is clean. Have your enema several hours prior to sex. Do not have an enema after sex. Frequent enemas can wash mucosa out of your rectum; do not do this daily! Never add stimulants like coffee or alcohol to enemas—you could become very ill. Never share enema equipment.

- *Relax!* Both the insertive and receptive partner need to be relaxed for successful anal penetration. Bathe together. Kiss and touch. Trade massages. Talk to each other. Share your anal sex fantasies. Feed your desire for anal play with each other.

I had the pleasure of introducing my girlfriend to her first anal experience. I tried to do it in the way that I would like to have had it done. I spooned her from the back, kissing her neck and rubbing whatever my hands could reach. After whispering in her ear what I was about to do to her, I began massaging her butt, working my way to her anus. I put plenty of lube on one finger of a gloved hand. I played with the outside for several minutes, all the while kissing her neck and talking to her. I asked her how it felt and whether I should continue. Finally, I inserted the tip of the finger. She was relaxed, not tense, no sharp intake of breath. I increased the penetration until I got about half of my finger in. We decided that that was enough. Since that time, almost two years ago, she has become more adventuresome, taking in whole fingers or a cute pink plug.

Finger Fucking

Your fingers are perfect tools for anal play—they're communicative, sensitive, and agile. As with vaginal penetration, you can use your fingers as a prelude to penetration with a dildo or hand, or as the main event.

Begin with your partner lying on her belly, with her legs open and her hips propped up on a pillow, or on her back with legs spread and a pillow under her butt. Slip on a latex glove and put some lube on your finger. Spread your partner's ass cheeks. With the palm of your hand facing up, run your lubed finger over the opening. Caress the anus with the pad of your finger; don't poke into the anus. Circle the opening slowly and then more quickly; and then run your finger across the opening. Watch her responses. Ask her what each stroke feels like. Build up a rhythm of touches and responses.

As the receptive partner, you are in charge. You can tell your partner exactly which touches you like and which you don't. You can ask her to slow down, to touch you with more or less pressure, or to add more lube to her finger. You may feel shy talking about your butt while a finger is stroking you. Or you may find it difficult to put words to such subtle physical sensations. Here's an opportunity to build up a vocabulary for anal sex. Soon you'll be telling your partner exactly how to stimulate your butt!

The insertive partner can put that information to good use. When the receptive partner indicates that a particular stroke is unpleasant—not enough lube, too hard, too scratchy—the insertive partner can watch for corresponding physical responses. Can you notice tension in the opening of your partner's anus? Has her anus closed? Are the muscles in her ass and thighs contracting? Do you notice a change in her breathing?

Similarly, when your partner is cooing with pleasure, notice how that translates into physical response. Can you notice her muscles relaxing? Has her anus opened? Is it contracting or pulsing with engorgement? Has the color of her anus deepened as blood fills the tissues? How's her breathing? What sounds is she making? Can you bring her to moans by gently caressing the anal opening with the pad of your finger?

Anal penetration combined with clitoral stimulation will make me come like a freight train!

You can ask her to instruct you as to exactly how to enter her. She may say, "Just the tip of your finger, please" or "Slide your finger in very slowly."

Draw your fingertip along the crack of her ass until the pad of your finger lies across her anal opening. Slip the pad of your finger into her. Enter her until just the tip of your finger is inside. Stay still until she adjusts to the pressure and fullness. As her internal sphincter muscles relax, her anus will seem roomier. Wait for her to tell you to insert more of your finger or to move inside her. She may like a subtle pulsing or fluttering of your fingertip; or she may prefer a subtle in-and-out motion.

When she's ready, push your finger in a little further—perhaps to the second knuckle. Again, stop and give her a chance to adjust to the sensations. Then push your finger all the way in. As necessary, pull your finger out and add more lube. Reenter slowly.

What if it hurts? If your partner feels pain, *stop*. Anal sex is not supposed to be painful. Pull out, lube up your finger, and start over. Caress the outside of the anus. Ask her to tell you when she'd like you to enter her again. Go slowly. But don't fill her as deeply—stop before you reach the point at which she felt pain. At each step of the way, let the receptive partner take the lead. As with vaginal penetration, give her just a little less than she seems to want. Let her desire grow to engulf your finger.

Once your finger is inside, ask her what kind of movement she likes. Experiment. You can circle the walls of her anus or rectum, or you can press against the front wall of her anus, providing indirect stimulation of her vagina, clitoris, and G-spot. You can gently thrust in and out. Remember that as you add more fingers, more fullness, more pressure, or try new strokes, you may need more lube.

Anal finger fucking is a slow build-up. She may want two or three fingers as her arousal increases. Or she may be satisfied with one. The first time you play anally, you may get no more than part of one finger inside her—that's fine. The goal is quality, not quantity.

Some women reach orgasm easily with anal penetration. The mounting pleasure in those ultrasensitive nerve endings radiates into an intense orgasm. If you prefer indirect clitoral stimulation, you may enjoy two fingers pressing rhythmically against the front wall of the rectum. That may be enough stimulation for your clitoris and G-spot. Or, you may like direct clitoral stimulation from fingers, a tongue, or a vibrator. You may like to be filled both vaginally and anally. Once you're fully aroused, you may like a hard thrusting motion, just remember to add plenty of lube.

Anal Fisting

Everything said about vaginal fisting applies tenfold to anal fisting, since the tissue of the rectum is less pliable and more easily torn than that of the vagina. Anal fisting requires patience, trust, and desire—and prodigious quantities of lube. Why would anyone want to put a whole hand into a partner's rectum—or feel her own anus and rectum stretched to receive a partner's hand? Like vaginal fisting, anal fisting is very intimate and intensely pleasurable.

Your anal fisting journey may begin one day when you feel sexually insatiable. Or, after a session of anal play, your partner may turn to you and say, "I felt so open, I swear I could've taken your whole hand."

Isn't anal fisting dangerous? Won't fisting stretch you out? No, fisting will *strengthen* your sphincters, not harm them. As one fisting devotee put it, "Training a muscle to do new and sometimes extraordinary things generally doesn't interfere with its function."[4] Tales of fisting enthusiasts wearing diapers are pure urban myth.

Anal fisting is a great activity for women who enjoy a long, slow session of anal play. You can't rush anal fisting. It also helps not to be goal oriented. Never force the body to accommodate more than feels pleasurable at the time. If you don't get a whole fist inside on the first try, you may on the next. Even if you never take an entire hand, you can have a lot of fun in the process of trying!

Fisting her anally is a huge rush. I am filled with aggression, yet am tender in my attempts.

As the receptive partner, you have to *want* your partner's hand inside you for your anus and rectum to open enough to receive it. You have to trust your partner not to hurt you—to know what she's doing—and to treat your openness and vulnerability with respect and caring.

As the insertive partner, you have to slow your desire down to the pace of your partner's responses. You have to want to feel your partner from the inside—badly enough to make an art of a practice few understand. You have to trust your partner to communicate at every step of the way.

As with all anal play, make sure your partner is aroused before you penetrate her. Begin with one or two fingers. Slowly increase the number of fingers until you have four fingers inserted up to the widest part of the hand. Add more lube frequently. As in vaginal fisting, when you meet resistance, pull back. Add lube. Resume, slowly. Your partner may like you to slide straight in or rotate your hand to twist your way in.

When you're inside, up to your wrist, be still until your partner adjusts to the intense sensations of fullness. She may want you to go no further, or she may ask for even deeper penetration. She may want you to gently rotate your hand, apply pressure on the front wall of the rectum, or thrust in and out—but by millimeters!

She may be too overwhelmed to even *think* of an orgasm—or she may feel an intense need to come and then have your hand out of her! You can stimulate her clitoris with your fingers, tongue, or a vibrator to bring her to orgasm. *Even if she demands that you remove your hand immediately, pull your hand gently and slowly out.*

Fisting is an overwhelmingly intense and vulnerable activity. Make sure you take time to care for each other after.

Strap-on Dildos

There's just something about being fucked in the ass with a dildo that really gets me hot. I like the way it make me feel vulnerable and open and used. Not politically correct lesbian stuff, I guess, but it's one of the best ways to make me orgasm.

Tristan Taormino's Beyond Our Bodies:
Emotional and Psychological Aspects of Anal Eroticism

Our emotional, psychological, and spiritual well-being plays a major role in our erotic experiences, and our experiences of anal sexuality are no exception.

People have a lot of fears and negative feelings about anal eroticism. Some of them stem from our society's myths and taboos about anal sex. Myths about anal sex being unnatural, perverted, dirty, painful, and dangerous have become very real fears in people's minds. It is important to realize that we are all made aware of the anal taboo and myths starting in childhood and therefore we are all affected in some way by them.

As the Receptive Partner, What Are Your Fears?

My lover will think I'm weird for wanting it.

I'll get hemorrhoids.

It will be messy, and my butt will smell bad.

I'll get constipated or have diarrhea.

It will hurt; something will get ruptured.

It won't feel good—I won't like it.

I won't be able to take her dildo.

I'll get an STD or another disease.

As the Insertive Partner, What Are Your Fears?

I'll hurt my partner or make her bleed.

It will be dirty, and I'll get shit on me.

I won't do it right.

I won't like it.

My lover will think I'm weird for wanting it.

I'll get an STD or another disease.

While most of these fears have their roots in myths and misconceptions about anal sex, it is important to respect and validate your partner when she shares her fears. Reassure each other that either one of you can stop activity at any time and be fully supported by the other one. Set concrete ground rules and boundaries about what is OK and what isn't; as experiences progress, the boundaries can change if needed. Each person needs to know that she will be safe from both pain and disease during anal sex and that there is mutual trust and respect.

Fear and tension that are not articulated and resolved will ultimately be felt in your anus, which will be tense and unwilling. Nina Hartley reminds us, "Of all the parts of your body, nothing knows a liar like your anus. So if your mind is saying 'Yes! Yes!' and your heart is saying 'No! No!' your anus will always listen to your heart." [5]

Having an open, honest discussion can help illuminate what each person wants from the experience and why, so that both people are less likely to make incorrect assumptions about the other person's desires and expectations. You can ask each other, What do you want? What do you expect? What are your needs and desires?

I want to work my way up to one finger, then stop.

I want to be able to have the small dildo in my butt.

I want everything to feel safe.

What have your previous experiences been with anal eroticism? Share them, discuss them. Why do you want to explore anal sensuality?

I want to explore something new with my partner.

I'm curious about what it feels like.

I've done it before and want to do it again.

You want to do it and I don't want to say no to you.

I want to feel closer to my lover.

It's something special and intimate and something I want to share with my partner.

I saw it in a porn movie, it turned me on, and I want to try it.

It's always been a fantasy of mine.

Fantasies can be incredibly powerful forces in our lives, erotic and otherwise. Many people fantasize about erotic activities like anal sex but are afraid to vocalize their desires. The myths and misinformation about anal sex contribute to the silence and sometimes prevent us from satisfying our curiosities. Sharing our sexual fantasies with a partner can deepen a sexual relationship and help us communicate our needs and desires.

It is equally important to distinguish our fantasies from our realities. If your favorite masturbatory fantasy involves someone ramming your butt repeatedly with a swollen silicone dick that makes you come every time, don't be surprised if you don't get the same result when you try it out. There are some fantasies that we can share and help bring to life and others that should probably remain fantasies. Have realistic expectations for yourself and know the limits of your own body, especially when it comes to anal sex. One finger in your anus and a whisper in your ear about that big dick might just do the trick.

During the experience, talk to each other, find out what feels good and what doesn't, what's working and what's not.

How does this feel?

Would you like more or less movement?

Do you want me to play with your pussy while I'm doing your ass?

How is this position?

That feels great—keep doing it.

I love doing this to you.

Do you want another finger now?

Afterward, have a little debriefing session to review how it went and get feedback you can use for next time. Remind each other about goals you set. Did I go too fast, did I use enough lube? Was there enough in-and-out movement, or do you want more of just that pressure feeling? What did you like about my fingers versus the butt plug? Is there something I can do differently next time? Do you want more genital stimulation while I'm playing with your butt? Compliments always feel good—criticism does not. Be generous when you communicate with your partner. If you want to tell her or him about something you didn't like, why not start that conversation with something you did like? But make sure you do talk about what wasn't pleasurable as well as what was pleasurable. Communication at all phases of an anal sex experience will ultimately enhance it, help both partners to articulate their needs, and, ideally, help everyone get what they want out of anal sex.

Having a big, tough dyke pound her enormous cock into your butt is a great fantasy—but in reality, you'd do best to start with fingers, working up to a small butt plug, then perhaps a slender dildo, to a wider plug, and finally a sizable dildo.

You might want to purchase a strap-on dildo just for anal play—not only is that hygienic (see "Anal Penetration—Safely" below), but you may find that though you like a thick, hefty dildo for vaginal play, you may be more comfortable with a long, slender dildo for anal play.

Receptive partner on top is a good position for anal sex with a strap-on dildo. The receptive partner can control the depth and speed of the thrusts. Rear entry can work well, too, if the insertive partner remains still as the receptive partner pushes back onto the dildo. The receptive partner stay in control, because the insertive partner doesn't have nerve endings in the tip of her dildo and the rectal tissue is easily torn. Remember that rectal tissue is much more delicate than vaginal tissue.

How-to's of Anal Penetration

- As the receptive partner, you're in charge. Tell your partner exactly how you want to be penetrated.
- Use lube—lots of lube. You can warm the lube by running hot water over the bottle before you play.
- Snap on a glove and lube up just one finger. Build up slowly.
- Circle the anus, stroking just the opening; kiss and nibble her inner thighs and ass as you caress her anus.
- Tease her—give her less than she wants, and then a little more.
- Slide the pad of your finger inside. Don't poke!
- Press toward the front or back of the rectum, move in circles inside her, thrust in and out.
- Slide a butt plug inside your partner—then penetrate her vaginally or stimulate her clitoris. (Position the tip of the plug beside her anus and enter her at at angle. Do not poke the plug into her.)
- With your dildo or fingers inside your partner, caress her breasts and belly.

- Climb on top of your partner and slowly lower yourself onto her dildo.
- Slide a vibrating cock ring over your dildo and grind against your partner's butt.
- On your hands and knees, push back against your partner's fingers or dildo.
- Bring out the toys—add nipple clamps, bondage, and vibrators to anal sex.
- Slip the fingers of one hand inside your partner's vagina while the other hand penetrates her anus.

Positions for Anal Penetration

The only time I've had an orgasm with anal penetration was when I was on my knees and my partner inserted her finger into my anus and slowly moved it in and out while I held a vibrator on my clitoris.

Any position that works for vaginal penetration can be adapted for anal play. You can kneel or sit between your partner's legs—a great position for finger fucking, fisting, or penetration with a hand-held dildo. Receptive partner on top is particularly useful for anal sex with a strap-on because the receptive partner can easily control the depth, speed, and intensity of her thrusts. Missionary position is also fine for strap-on anal sex. Many anal sex aficionados prefer missionary position in a sling to any other anal sex position. Side by side will work for more gentle and slow penetration.

Rear entry is a favorite position for anal finger fucking, fisting, and strap-on sex. This position allows the receptive partner a lot of movement; if the insertive partner remains still, she can completely control the action.

Toys for Anal Penetration

Once again, lube tops the shopping list. When it comes to anal penetration, lubricant is the most important item in your toy chest. Unlike the vagina, the rectum is *not* self-lubricating. And the tissue of the rectum, while elastic, is fragile and easily torn.

Many women switch to oil-based lubes, like Crisco, for anal play. Oil-based lubes do not evaporate as quickly as water-based lubes. They are thicker and more viscous and create a more slippery feel. Some find that mixing olive oil with their favorite thick water-based lube will make a slipperier concoction.

However, I encourage the use of water-based lubricant for two reasons: First, if, despite your best efforts, should lube drip from the anus into the vagina, the use of oil-based lube will make a bad situation worse. No only will you get anal bacterial in your vagina, but the oil will help it stay there. Second, petroleum products break down latex, causing small perforations in condoms and gloves.

Can you use oil-based lube safely for anal penetration? Yes, but with care. First, take extra precautions to make sure lube doesn't drip from the anus into the vagina. Second, change your glove every 15 minutes. The oil will not degrade the latex in your glove in less than 15 minutes. Condoms, however, are much thinner than latex gloves; if you use oil-based lube with a latex condom, assume that you will have to disinfect the toy after use—since the oil will have made pinprick holes in the condom. If you really want to use an oil-based lube with your dildo, invest in polyurethane condoms. (*Never* use oil-based lube on a latex condom covering a penis—after coming in contact with petroleum in the lube, the condom will offer you no protection.)

Nitrile gloves—in addition to being useful for people with latex allergies— can be used safely with oil-based lube.

There are a few basic rules for choosing toys for anal penetration:

- The toy must have a flared base to prevent it from slipping inside your rectum and working its way into the colon. Anal beads must be securely fastened to their string and have a ring on the end to hold onto.
- The toy must have a smooth surface—no sharp edges or breakable parts.
- You must be able to clean the toy with antibacterial soap and hot water.
- If you intend to use the toy to penetrate your partner deeply, it must be flexible enough to maneuver the curves of the rectum.

Many toys used for vaginal penetration, such as dildos and harnesses, work well for anal penetration. There are also toys designed specifically for anal play. Butt plugs are designed to stay inside the rectum. They take advantage of the sphincter muscles' tendency to grip around an object. Butt plugs range in size from a few inches long and no thicker than your thumb to bigger than a fist. You can even find butt plugs shaped like star fruit. You can purchase a variety of vibrating butt plugs as well.

Anal beads are small balls attached to a string. During anal play, you insert the progressively larger orbs into your partner's rectum. When she's about to come, you pull them out. Traditionally, anal beads were made from cheap hard plastic and even had sharp seams that had to be filed down. Now you can find anal beads in a variety of materials, including silicone, which is much softer and more hygienic (you can boil silicone to clean it).

There are a number of vibrators designed for anal insertion, including a long, slender, curving vibrator with a flexible spine that allows it to retain any shape you bend it to.

Don't forget to start small! Buy the smaller butt plug; you can always move on to something larger later on. See Chapter 15, "Sex Toys and Accoutrements," for more on penetrative toys.

Anal Penetration—Safely

The number one safety rule for anal penetration is: *If it hurts, stop!* Don't engage in any activity that could possibly abrade the lining of the rectum. Don't continue any activity that causes bleeding.

Why would a lesbian need to wear a latex glove for anal sex? No semen, no problem—right? Wrong! If you have small cuts on your fingers, you could be infected by your partner's *E. coli* bacteria.[6] Before you toss out the gloves, pour some vinegar over your hand. If you have any small cuts, you'll know!

Don't share toys without thoroughly cleaning them with disinfectant soap and hot water. Even if you use a condom on that dildo, clean it before you use it on yourself or another partner. Always clean toys after anal sex and before vaginal penetration, to prevent anal bacteria from getting inside your vagina. If possible, buy silicone toys, which you can clean by boiling for two or three minutes. Or, keep a set of "dedicated" anal toys.

Safer Anal Penetration

- Get a manicure. Make sure your nails are smoothly filed.

- Use latex, nitrile, or vinyl gloves.

- Put on a fresh glove when you switch activities or partners.

- Use water-based lube.

- Use condoms on your dildos. Always use a fresh condom when switching sexual activities or partners.

- Don't share dildos and vibrators without cleaning in between uses.

- Don't allow bacteria from the anus to enter the vagina.

Where to Learn More

You may be lucky enough to find an anal sex workshop at a sex-toy boutique near you. If not, check out the relatively new instructional videos on anal sex—see the "Resources" section for videos by Tristan Taormino, Shar Rednour, and Nina Hartley.

A search for anal fisting information on the Web turned up a number of sites for gay men. When it comes to sexually explicit content, lesbians have a long history of borrowing from gay men. Perhaps by the time of the next edition of this book, there will be lesbian-specific information on the Web about anal fisting. For now, I highly recommend RedRight, a web site that takes its name from the hanky code. A red hanky in the right back pocket indicates that one is a fisting "bottom" (receptive partner). See below.

Suggested Web Link:

RedRight

www.winternet.com/~redright/fffaq.htm

NOTES

1. Toys in Babeland web site, www.babeland.com
2. Robert Morgan, quoted by Tristan Taormino in *The Ultimate Guide to Anal Sex for Women* (Cleis Press, 1997), 88.
3. Jack Morin, *Anal Pleasure and Health* (Down There Press, 1998), 227–29. According to Morin, hemorrhoids are caused by tension in the internal sphincter muscles, along with a diet of overly refined foods. "[W]hen rectal entry is accomplished through relaxation, the results are beneficial, even to the hemorrhoid sufferer."
4. RedRight web site, www.winternet.com/~redright/fffaq.htm
5. Nina Hartley, "Nina Hartley's Guide to Anal Sex" (Adam and Eve Productions, 1994).
6. Ask Dr. Myrtle, A Woman's Touch web site, www.a-womans-touch.com

SOURCE OF SIDEBAR

Tristan Taormino, "Beyond Our Bodies: Emotional and Psychological Aspects of Anal Eroticism" from *The Ultimate Guide to Anal Sex for Women* by Tristan Taormino. (Cleis Press, 1997).

chapter twelve

Gender (Not Destiny)

Lesbian sex begins and ends with who I am as a woman.

GENDER IS SEXY. That lesbian in heels and hose is so unmistakably feminine and so aggressively erotic—and so unconditionally interested in her own sex. That butch exudes sexual confidence—standing with thumbs hooked in belt loops, flexing her thigh muscles to draw attention to the lump in her jeans. That ambiguously gendered person is at once hotly erotic and so startling as to be disturbing.

For some, gender is a plaything, the best sex toy in the play room. They enjoy cross-dressing and purposely mixing gender signifiers—femmes with dicks, butches in high femme drag. For others, gender's a matter of style, a way of presenting oneself to the world. And for still other, words like "butch," "femme," "queer," and "transgender"—and even "androgyny"—speak to a deeply held identity, one that can't be peeled off at the end of the night like a costume.

Whether a dildo is just a dildo is up to you, of course. How you relate to gender is personal—and no one's opinion of your gender matters but your own. You needn't locate yourself on a gender continuum of masculinity and femininity or label yourself at all unless that's useful for you.

Your gender identity can shift and change over the course of a lifetime. Or, your gender identity may remain constant—but your acceptance of yourself, your capacity to be on the outside exactly who you are on the inside, may grow over the years.

What does gender have to do with lesbian sex? Think of your "sex" as your physical equipment, your "gender" as what you do with it, and your "sexual orientation" as the territory of your desire.

What Is Gender?

How do you know you're female? Are you female because you have a clitoris? Because your adult life has been marked by cycles of ovulation and menstruation? Because you were raised as a girl? Because you were forced to be female? Because you "feel" female?

Gender is more than anatomical sex; gender is how you relate to your biological sex. Your gender identity may or may not agree with your biological sex. For instance, you may have a woman's body and identify as male. You may experience your clitoris as a cock, your breasts as a chest.

You may have a woman's body and delight in your femininity—yet know to the core of your being that your experience of the feminine bears little resemblance to that of a heterosexual woman. The distinctions may be beyond words.

You may find all of the outward signals of gender irrelevant—your woman's body speaks for itself. You may view yourself as androgynous. Or you may prefer to skip the discussion entirely.

You may be anatomically male and identify as female. On you, a penis is your clitoris; a prostate, your G-spot. Regardless of how you're "read" on the street, you know you're female.

So, then, what makes a person female or male? Is it anatomy? Identity? Some combination of the two?

Gender roles can be defined by fashion (who wears the pants), economics (who gets the paycheck), and sexual roles (who's on top), as well as the particulars of culture and religion, history and class. (Remember when Rosie the Riveter was expected to morph into Donna Reed? "No more power tools for *you*, honey!")

You may try to "read" gender by observing secondary sex characteristics, such as facial structure and facial hair, fat and muscle distribution, body mass, vocal pitch, movement, and linguistic style.

You can determine "sex" anatomically by looking at the external genitalia. Historically, women were defined as nonmales (penis = male; no penis = female). You can look, instead, to reproductive biology: a female has ovaries, a male testes. You can examine hormones, defining a female as a person who produces more estrogen and progesterone than testosterone. You can look at genetics, defining a female as a person with XX rather than XY chromosomes.

Male and female sexual anatomy is actually quite similar—we share the same bits of engorging, erectile tissue and the same nerve endings. We're simply arranged differently. In the early stages of fetal development, there is no anatomic difference between male and female. The genitals begin to differentiate at about the eighth week.[1] Glans tissue develops into either the glans of the clitoris or the glans of the penis. Clitoral hood and foreskin develop from identical tissue, as do the labia and scrotum, the testes and ovaries, and the shaft of the penis and the shaft of the clitoris. It isn't until the fifth month of pregnancy that you can reliably detect a fetus's sex from an ultrasound procedure.

Intersexuality

But what if all gender characteristics aren't in alignment? In fact, according to the Intersex Society of North America (ISNA), 1 infant in 500 is born with something other than XX or XY chromosomes.[2] Intersexed infants may have genitals that don't appear distinctly male or female. So who's to decide whether that genital appendage is a clitoris or a penis?

Unfortunately, medical authorities consider it their prerogative to make that decision. A baby's phallus must be a minimum of 1 inch long to be considered a penis; however, a clitoris must *not* be longer than $^3/_8$ of an inch. That leaves more than $^1/_2$ inch of what one writer calls "a veritable pubic Twilight Zone, the land of ambiguous genitalia."[3] What happens to the infant born with a phallus longer than $^3/_8$ of an inch but shorter than 1 inch?

The medical response to intersex conditions has been to intervene surgically—in some cases soon after birth and in other cases at puberty (when unexpected sexual development may occur). Most intersex infants are determined to be female: the overly large clitoris is surgically reduced to a "normal" size. As a result of such mutilation,[4] many intersex women have reduced clitoral sensitivity, and some are unable to reach orgasm.

The rationale for early medical intervention is that what a child doesn't know won't hurt her—which, of course, is anything but true. The real reason behind most surgery on intersexed children is discomfort with the idea that "male" and "female" might be something other than immutable categories.

Not surprisingly, human variation doesn't fit into those two neat little boxes. According to the ISNA, "Anatomic sex differentiation occurs on a male/female continuum."[5]

Yet the medical approach to intersexuality is rooted in the idea that to function "successfully" in society, children must have a "fixed" gender identity from an early age. The child's genitals must "match the standard anatomy" for his or her gender. Boys must have penises, and girls must have vaginas "with no easily noticeable phallus."[6]

Are intersex women lesbian? Bisexual? Heterosexual? Can you tell by looking at a person's genitals if she or he is intersexed? What pronouns do intersexed people prefer? All of this will vary from person to person. Ask.

I'm transgendered due to an intersex birth condition, a dyke, and femme by nature. Thank the Goddess we are more than the adjectives we and society use to identify us!

Transgender and Transsexual

"Transgender" is an umbrella term that includes all who don't feel that their designated sex (female or male) exactly matches their gender identity. This can include male-to-female transsexuals (MTF) and female-to-male transsexuals (FTM), along with transvestites, drag kings and drag queens, and even butches and femmes who view their experience of being "female" as different from the dominant social construct.

Some people think of their gender on a continuum, so butch lesbians may identify strongly with female-to-male transsexuals, both of whom are quite conscious of their own degree of masculinity—though one carries a driver's license that says "female" and the other "male."

A transsexual is a person whose intent is to live as a gender other than that assigned at birth. Most transsexuals engage in some process of altering primary and secondary sexual characteristics, through hormone treatment or surgery or both. Some transsexuals live full time in their chosen gender without any alteration of physiology. They don't feel that they must alter their physical bodies to match conventional definitions of male and female. Others engage in hormone treatment without any intention of undergoing genital reconstructive surgery—because the surgery is very expensive and the results are often less than optimal. Transsexuals can be homosexual, bisexual, or heterosexual, and may identify as either butch or femme. They may wish to pass as just another man or just another woman—or they may identify as transsexual or "third gender." Regardless, male-to-female transsexuals are women and female-to-male trans-sexuals are men.

Gender reassignment can affect sex drive. Many MTFs in transition experience a drop in sex drive when they begin taking estrogen, and many FTMs notice a sharp increase in sex drive when they begin taking testosterone. But the hormonally driven changes in libido are only half the story. Greeting the world as a newly formed person is no small challenge—remember puberty?

Male-to-Female Transsexuals

I am a woman who happened to be born male through no fault of her own.

Hormonal treatment for male-to-female transsexuals involves taking anti-androgen and estrogen, which results in a decreasing of male secondary sex characteristics and an increasing of female sexual characteristics: less body hair,

---

I love breasts and a dick on the same body.

less muscle mass, higher-pitched voice, growth of breasts, softening of the skin, rounding of the hips, and the development of a girlish tush!

Surgical techniques include upper-body surgery to enlarge breasts (though many MTFs find estrogen enhances their breasts quite adequately) and lower-body surgeries to reshape the male genitalia into a clitoris and vagina.

Lower-body surgery techniques include vaginoplasty and labioplasty. In one technique, the penis is inverted to create a vagina, which is then lined with skin from the penis and scrotum. So while the new vagina isn't self-lubricating, it *is* made of tissue that engorges with sexual arousal. Some surgeons utilize tissue from the glans of the penis to create a clitoris capable of sensation. They may also construct a cervix from the tissue of the glans of the penis. [7]

Some MTFs report that they have difficulty reaching orgasm once estrogen and anti-androgens render their penis nonfunctional. They must learn to experience arousal and orgasm in an entirely new way.

> *When I transitioned, I became friends with a bisexual girl. Since the hormone regime I was taking meant that my male genitalia no longer functioned, she taught me to experience pleasure in other ways. I had my first female orgasm, and I've never looked back.*

Female-to-Male Transsexuals

> *Becoming comfortable with my body has allowed me to enjoy sex more. I haven't physically changed my body yet, but knowing that I will has freed me somehow.*

For female-to-male transsexuals, hormonal treatment involves taking testosterone, resulting in increased body hair and muscle mass, deepening of vocal pitch, loss of those curves, and, often, increased sex drive. Surgical techniques include upper-body surgery to reshape the chest and lower-body surgeries to reshape the female genitals into a penis and scrotum.

Testosterone produces an enlarged clitoris for many FTMs. The clitoris can grow to as much as three inches long. Some FTMs further enhance the clitoris by pumping it up with a nipple pump (a device that can be found in sex shops catering to gay men). A three-inch erect clitoris can be inserted into the slit in the base of a dildo designed to hold an egg vibrator.

Some FTMs experience a male sex drive distinct from their sense of their sexuality prior to using testosterone. They speak of an urgency to reach orgasm unlike anything they had previously known.

Upper-body surgery involves a double mastectomy and reshaping of the nipples to produce a flat, masculine chest. Some FTMs find that gender reassignment surgery rekindles an interest in nipple play. Once the physical shape of the chest fits their gender identity, they may find that where once they preferred to ignore their breasts, they now like their nipples tweaked, pinched, sucked, or bitten. Of course, interest in nipple play will vary from person to person.

Lower-body surgery techniques include vaginectomy, metaoidioplasty, and phalloplasty. Vaginectomy is removal of the vagina. In metaoidioplasty, the testosterone-enhanced clitoris is surgically freed from the surrounding structure and the tissue of the labia is used to create a scrotal sac. Phalloplasty involves construction of a penis using skin grafts from other parts of the body. Some procedures involve implanting inflatable prostheses for erection. Some FTMs also opt for complete hysterectomies.[8]

Many female-to-male transsexuals don't opt for genital reconstruction and so, physiologically, remain female—though they'd hardly wish to be called "women"! These transgendered men have a testosterone-enhanced clitoris, facial and body hair, and increased musculature—but they also have a vagina, a G-spot, and a cervix. Many identify as "queer" or bisexual, rather than as lesbian.

Partners of Transgendered Women and Men

"What pronouns should I use to address my transsexual friends?" "If I date a preop MTF, does that mean I'm bisexual?" "What if her driver's license says she's female?" "Can I bring my FTM partner to a women-only party?" "My lesbian friends are acting as if I'm a traitor. Help!"

When your lovers and friends begin the process of questioning gender identity, most likely you'll have a few questions of your own! Thankfully, significant others of transgendered people have begun to organize resources, including e-mail discussion lists and support groups. Contact any of the trans-gender support organizations listed in the "Resources" for more information—and check out the Web links at the end of this chapter.

My current long-term primary partner identifies as FTM. I think this has had a role in my bisexual identity.

So what pronouns should you use? The ones your transgendered partner requests of you, of course! Can you be sexual with a transgendered partner and identify as a lesbian? Some female partners of FTMs identify as bisexual or queer rather than lesbian—if nothing else, they feel it's supportive of a partner who no longer identifies as a woman and therefore can't be in a lesbian relationship. What you call yourself, however, is up to you. Sexual orientation is a personal matter. (See "Sexual Orientation," below.)

The most femme dyke I ever slept with was an MTF transsexual. It was rough, though—I found that I spent a lot of time defending her.

A quick glance at the listings of organizations in the "Resource" section will reveal many different ways of defining "woman-only" space: genetic women only; genetic and transsexual women; genetic women, and transgendered women living full-time (24/7) as women; those having XX chromosomes or living as women 24/7; lesbians and bisexual women; genetic women, FTMs in transition, and transgendered women; genetic females (irrespective of gender expression) and MTFs (irrespective of genital surgery); woman and trans men; and anyone who identifies as a woman.

Sexual Orientation

Are you a lesbian because you desire women—or because you don't desire men? Are you bisexual if you fantasize about having sex with men? If you *have* sex with men?

Many of us are familiar with the Kinsey scale, which offers a way of looking at sexual orientation on a 0 to 6 scale, with 0 representing exclusively heterosexual behavior, 6 representing exclusively homosexual behavior, and 3 representing bisexual behavior. Forward-thinking though he was at the time, Alfred Kinsey devised this continuum in 1948!

Kinsey was looking at his respondents' behavior. Sexual orientation is, of course, far more complex than which sex acts you perform with which partners. Whom do you desire? Who stirs your fantasies? Whom do you love? For instance, on the Kinsey scale, a lesbian who comes out in midlife after 20 years of heterosexual marriage would probably rank somewhere between heterosexual and bisexual—even though she longed for sex with women for many of those 20 years, rarely enjoyed sex with her husband, delights in her new sex life, and intends never to have sex with a man again!

Playing with the Boys

Imagine for a moment two women with identical sexual histories. One calls herself a lesbian, the other a bisexual. How is this possible? Sexual orientation is a matter of self-identification—labels others may toss onto you have little bearing on your realities. For some women, being bisexual means that they enjoy sex with both men and women equally. For others, it means that they feel they have the potential to fall in love with a person of either gender. Some women are sexual with both men and women for their entire lives without labeling themselves at all. You may have sex with men, yet feel that the term "lesbian" best describes who you are and whom you most desire.

*Aspects of my erotic life with
men get incorporated into my sex with women—
I am unable to separate the two.*

Many women enjoy sex with partners who are as queer as they are! Your preferences may run to gay and bisexual men, or to transsexuals of all genders and in all stages of transition. The sex you have with men and women may be qualitatively very different. For instance, you may enjoy strapping on a dildo to penetrate a male partner, but enjoy being penetrated by your woman lover—or vice versa. You may enjoy nearly identical sex acts with partners of either sex. The sexual activities, roles, or styles you like may vary from person to person and have nothing to do with gender at all.

Perhaps you prefer to be sexual with women whose sexual orientation matches your own. What if you're a lesbian who wants to have sex exclusively with women who also have sex exclusively with women? That's fine. State your preferences without apology—but remember, yours is a preference, *not* a moral position.

Butch/Femme

Many lesbians and bisexual women find that the dynamics of butch/femme attraction intensifies sex. The gender contrast between two women sparks a *frisson* that's very exciting. Some butches prefer "high" femmes as partners—whether they be powerful femmes fatales or cherished submissives. Some femmes may even prefer FTMs as partners, appreciating such a high degree of masculinity in someone who wasn't born and raised male.

The terms "butch" and "femme" may describe your gender identity as much as your sexuality. For you, butch/femme is not just about romance and fashion—or, for that matter, who's on top. After all, a femme is a femme—whether or not there is a butch in the vicinity. Her gender identity is her own, requiring no validation from her complement. Similarly, a butch is a butch regardless of whether a femme takes her arm.

What butch/femme sexuality means varies from person to person. Butches and femmes come in all genders and sexual orientations. You may enjoy butch-on-butch sex or femme-to-femme sex. You may find that you enjoy playing with gender signifiers—like hair, clothing, sexual apparatus, and roles—without

10 Myths About Butch/Femme

1. *All bi girls are femme.* Not so. Some very hot, tough butches identify as bisexual.

2. *Butches are stronger than femmes. Masculine = strong; feminine = weak. Butch = top; femme = bottom.* If you believe this, go straight to your room and don't come out until you have read Simone de Beauvoir's *The Second Sex*.

3. *Butches don't cry.* See #2. 'Nuff said.

4. *You have to locate yourself somewhere on the butch/femme continuum. Femmy butch. Butchy femme. Tomboy. Boychick. Butch. Femme.* Nope! You're not required to label yourself. And if you identify one way now, that may not be your lifelong identity. Gender can change over time.

5. *Real butches don't get penetrated. Well, maybe in the ass. But if you eroticize your female genitals, you're not really butch.* No way. Many butches love vaginal penetration—with fingers, dildos, and fists. And, while we're on the subject, not all femmes like penetrative sex. And some butches love it.

6. *Femmes don't wear power tools.* Some femmes strap a dildo on and love to penetrate their lovers. Personally, I find nothing hotter than a beautiful woman with a surprise under her skirt.

7. *All femmes wear lipstick. And heels, garters, and lacy lingerie.* Not necessarily so! Lots of women identify as femme without any interest in traditional girl gear. Femme is about sexuality and gender—not necessarily fashion.

8. *Butches are big and femmes are small.* Butches and femmes come in all shapes and sizes. Butches can have 40DD tits and femmes can wear training bras— or no bra at all!

9. *All butches play sports.* Not true. Some butches play the piano. And some butches would rather go shopping than play football.

10. *All butches are attracted to femmes and vice versa.* Lots of butches date other butches. And many femmes love femmes.

---

adopting a full-time butch or femme identity. You don't have to fit a certain body type or personality style to identify as butch or femme. You needn't wear makeup to be femme or change the oil on your truck to be butch—or adhere to any other gender stereotypes you may have spent years trying to escape. Think of butch/femme as a way of looking at how gender shows up in your life. Butch/femme is a potent sexual dynamic. It's *yours* to create.

From packing and penetration to passing, lesbians have much to say about butch/femme sexual dynamics.

There is something so sexy when the feminine gender is mixed with that masculine finish. A butch woman makes me swoon.

I love the exchange of power that goes back and forth from butch to femme. As a butch, I protect my femme partner from harm and am dominant in sex. Yet, at the same time, I am a willing servant to my femme's desires, putting her needs and wishes before mine.

When I walk, my hips swish and my breasts bounce and my thighs roll with the fluidity that is my femininity.

High femme is not an everyday thing. But when I go out to cruise or party, it borders on the drag-queenly. This excites me—and attracts butches with balls!

While I am very pleased to be a woman, my body is read as a heterosexual one because of the way I live in it, move in it, and adorn it. I don't like that. But it's the femme conundrum.

I am a transgendered stone butch and it is crucial that my lover respect my body image. I have a female body but like to be touched in a way that honors my masculinity.

I prefer for my butch to "run the fuck." I love the feeling of lying in my lover's arms as she ravishes me! It thrills me to see the love and lust in her eyes as she makes love to me.

*I like it when butches pack.
It shows me they're forward-thinking
and well-prepared. Good form!*

Sometimes, when my femme has orgasmed many, many times, I lie with my head down by her cunt and use a vibrator, imagining it as my dick. Both of us find this very hot and I have powerful orgasms this way.

I am sassy and willful and not easy to "take down" sexually. I need the authority, confidence, and uncompromising identity of a stone butch. Being a stone femme means that I do not want a sex partner who expects a 50/50 sexual relationship (she gets me off and then I get her off). If a butch softens when she's with me and lets me touch her genitals and breasts without re-signifying them as male parts, then I most likely would not want to be with that person sexually again.

I adore only feminine women—and men, for that matter!

Suggested Web links:

BUTCH-FEMME.COM
> www.butch-femme.com

THE INTERSEX SOCIETY OF NORTH AMERICA (ISNA)
> www.isna.org

FTM INTERNATIONAL, INC.
> www.ftm-intl.org

INTERNATIONAL FOUNDATION FOR GENDER EDUCATION
> www.ifge.org

SOFFA USA
SIGNIFICANT OTHERS, FRIEND, FAMILY OR ALLY OF TRANSGENDERED PERSONS
> members.aol.com/SOFFAUSA/

NOTES

1. Cheryl Chase, correspondence, September 1999.

2. ISNA web site, www.isna.org

3. Annalee Newitz, "When Doctors Try to Fix What Ain't Broke," GettingIt.com, July 27, 1999, www.gettingit.com

4. Like other clitoridectomies performed for cultural or religious reasons, surgery performed on intersex children amounts to genital mutilation. Thanks to intersex activists, such medical practices are changing in some areas.

5. ISNA web site, www.isna.org

6. Alice Domurat Dreger, "'Ambiguous sex'—or Ambivalent Medicine?" *Hastings Center Report*, vol. 28, no. 3, 24–35, May/June 1998. The full text of the article can be found on the ISNA web site, www.isna.org

7. Transgender Surgical and Medical Care Center, web site, www.tsmccenter.com

8. Ibid.

chapter thirteen

Play Nice! (...or Else)

I don't think all sex is about power, but playing with power in sex has taught me a lot about power in the "real" world.

DO YOU FANTASIZE ABOUT BINDING A PARTNER'S WRISTS AND ANKLES TO THE bedposts? Do you thrill to the notion of being helplessly bound? Perhaps your fantasies feature sensory deprivation—facilitated by blindfolds, hoods, body bags, gags, or elaborate bondage. Your tastes may run to erotic torture, denying and permitting your partners' orgasms as you wish ("Ask me nicely." *"Please!"* "No. Ask me again..."). You may employ sensual implements such as feathers and fur-covered paddles—or wield implements more traditionally associated with "heavy" S/M play, such as whips, crops, and canes. Your body may show permanent markings from cutting or branding.

Sadomasochism, dominance and submission, edge play, power exchange, and sensual magic are all names for a kind of sex play that involves the consensual transfer of power between partners. People use the term "S/M" to refer to a wide range of sexuality whether or not it really involves sadism and/or masochism. BDSM is an umbrella term combining bondage, dominance and submission, and sadomasochism.

Not all BDSM play involves pain—some devotees play for years with nary a bruise. Their interests are in dominance and submission, sensory deprivation, and sensation play. You can be extremely sadistic without laying a hand on your partner (what could be more sadistic?). And not all BDSM players engage in the role-play of dominance and submission; some folks simply enjoy a good, hard whipping.

What all BDSM players have in common, though, is that they use this edgy form of sexuality to push their comfort zone and discover something about themselves. They are investigating an area of human sexuality that may be scary and overwhelming in its intensity, yet can yield pleasures unattainable by other means. It's most certainly taboo.

Why would you choose to play with dominance and submission, sadism and masochism, sensory deprivation, or physical pain in the context of sex? Well, because kinky sex is hot, of course! Many women find that dancing between safety and danger turns them on.

Ouch!!! (Yum...)

Why would someone like pain? Isn't that sick? Not at all! The human nervous system has the capacity to process a huge range of sensations. Whether those sensations are experienced as pleasure or pain is a subjective matter.

Have you ever discovered "love bites" on your neck the morning after a particularly passionate night of sex—and wondered just when they occurred? You may find that when you're sexually aroused, you thrill to sensations that under other circumstance you'd find annoying or intolerable. When you're sufficiently turned on, a twist of the nipple or a bite on the inner thigh may, in fact, heighten your arousal.

The line separating pain and pleasure can get quite thin once your endorphins kick in. Endorphins are hormone-like chemicals released by your brain when the body is under stress or in pain. Runners speak of attaining a state of bliss when they push themselves beyond their perceived limits. You can get an endorphin high at the gym, during sex, or while energetically wielding a flogger in a long S/M scene. And you can get an endorphin high while experiencing pain.

Like opiates, endorphins don't make the pain go away, but they make you feel awfully good while it's happening! Under the right circumstances, you may be able to ride wave after wave of pain, breathing into the sensations as they radiate

What Is BDSM?

B&D	**Bondage and Discipline**
D/S	**Dominance and Submission**
S/M	**Sadism and Masochism**

through your body. In fact, you may astonish yourself by requesting another and another and another....

> *There's an eroticism to a rhythmic beating. The repetitive thud of a whip can translate directly into clitoral pulses....*

What are the right circumstances for getting blissed-out on pain? Naturally, response to pain will vary from person to person. Here are some common ways to manipulate pain in BDSM play:

- *Warm up.* A gentle warm-up will help make your scene last. Begin with very light strokes, continuing until your partner's buttocks or shoulders show a nice warm glow. A sensual whipping—in which no single stroke of the lash exceeds your partner's perceived pain threshold—will leave her ready for something more intense.
- *Pacing.* Let your partner recover from one sensation before going on to the next. Intermittent hard beating, mixing sensual strokes with sharper strokes, will also help her take more pain and stretch her limits (if she so desires). After a painful blow, place the palm of your hand at the point of contact. Soothe the rising welt or mark with the warmth of your body.
- *Breathing.* Breathe *into* the sensations; don't hold your breath or tense your muscles *against* the pain. Ride with it.
- *Sensation.* Some women prefer thud to sting—or vice versa. Different toys produce different sensations. Generally, the thinner the toy, the more stinging its sensations. So a wide paddle or heavy flogger will produce a "thuddier" sensation than a thin rod or single-tailed whip. Some women who

love the deep pounding of a heavy whip seem to be able to take it forever; others prefer the discrete, searing lines of pain laid down by an expert caning.

- *Erotic context.* Many women find they can take more pain when the context is eroticized. You may find that a finger slowly stroking your clitoris will more than ameliorate the pain of that strap on your butt!
- *Discipline and reward.* In some scenes, pain is a reward for a good deed; in others, it's delivered as punishment for a mistake, real or imagined.
- *Submission.* Some women may find they can eroticize pain in the context of a dominance and submission scene. Simply put, they wish to please their top, and if the top enjoys administering a good beating, they aim to take it!
- *Masochism.* Finally, a masochist craves pain in the context of an S/M scene. Even when pain isn't accompanied by erotic touching, and regardless of whether she gives a hoot about pleasing her top or whether the pain is being administered as punishment or reward, she may simply desire pain's sensations.

Negotiation

As a top, I like to ask the bottom to pick the toys she likes best, plus one she would hate to feel. I love the physical act of flogging, the swing and rhythm of both bodies giving and receiving. Paddling as well, if only to have a woman on her knees or over my lap. I would have to say orgasm denial is my all-time favorite activity. The rewards are lovely.

Negotiating an S/M scene involves exploring each partner's desires, needs, limits, and safety concerns to find a common ground from which to proceed. The keys to negotiation are honesty and mutual respect. Negotiation is *not* about persuasion.

Negotiation is an art all its own. You can negotiate a specific scene or an entire relationship. You can negotiate at a café over coffee, over the phone, or via e-mail. You can even stop a scene to renegotiate a particular aspect of play. Longstanding partners may negotiate a scene in five minutes, while new partners may spend weeks discussing the details of a proposed scene. In fact, the anticipation may be half the fun!

10 Benefits of BDSM Play

1. Kink is hot! Many women enjoy intense orgasms after a prolonged session of S/M play.

2. You can dance between pleasure and pain and enjoy an endorphin high.

3. You can let go of control—or take control. Few of us have safe or consensual opportunities in the daily grind to give up or take control.

4. You can play with dynamics that wouldn't be safe or even desirable in "real" life. You wouldn't really want to rape your girlfriend or be humiliated by your closest friends—yet playing with these may turn you on like nothing else.

5. You can take risks. For the thrill seeker, an S/M scene is like a three-hour roller coaster ride. Sure, you're strapped in, but nevertheless you are hurtling toward the earth in an open car! You'll not lack for thrills when you find yourself tied to a post in a basement dungeon as a hooded woman approaches wielding a long, thin whip....

6. You can surrender your fears and revel in that shadow side of yourself you've done so well to keep hidden! "I never knew I could be so mean!" "I didn't know I would feel so, well, serene on my hands and knees polishing a pair of boots!"

7. You can strip away the armor of daily life. "Pain and humiliation move me to a raw place where I can access my genuine self, without fear or hesitation," wrote one woman.

8. You can experience healing and catharsis in letting go and trusting yourself (and your partner) at such a core level.

9. You can experience heightened intimacy with your partner as you embark on an erotic adventure together.

10. You may discover a spiritual component in the transcendence of everyday concerns, the quest for self-transformation, and the ritual of an S/M scene.

Many women say they learned more about healthy boundaries from S/M negotiation than from any support group or self-help book. Negotiating an S/M scene puts in stark relief the kind of self-denial that often masquerades as "politeness." To negotiate an S/M scene, you must know what you want and be willing to name it. You're expected to state your desires in detail and without justification, and to say no to anything you don't want—no explanation necessary. You're expected to take care of your wants and needs and let your partner take care of hers.

For many women, the open communication required in scene negotiation is a relief from the unspoken demands and contracts that can creep into many relationships ("If I do X for you, you'll do Y for me"). As one woman wrote, "I prefer to have my power exchange up front and out on the table."

So how *do* you negotiate a scene? Scene negotiation is best conducted between equals (not in top/bottom roles) and outside of a sexual context. Everyone has a favorite method. You can pull out your Erotic Play list from Chapter 2, "Desire and Fantasy," and mark each item "yes," "no," or "maybe." Your choices can be good for a day, for a month, or for one particular scene with one particular partner. You can begin by asking yourself (and your partner) a few basic questions:

What type of scene are you interested in? Do you fantasize elaborate role-play with costumes and props—Mutiny on the *Bounty?* Or perhaps genteel torture in a Victorian boarding school scene? Would you like to be tied to a whipping post and flogged in front of six of your friends?

What are your essential ingredients for a hot scene? Is bondage essential? An exquisite collection of S/M toys? What about orgasm? A woman who plays as a submissive bottom wrote, "I want to be fully recognized. I want to give myself up to someone else for the pure pleasure of having her be completely attentive to and conscious of me."

What are your limits? Will you take a paddle? A cane? What about blood play?

Is it OK to leave bruises? "I get off on seeing the marks I've left," wrote one woman. "I'm impressed by the body's reactions, the redness, swelling, and bruising. I like to admire my work the next day."

I like the loss of control.
I like being in my top's hands and,
in theory at least, not being able to get away.

What are the things you might like to try? "I fantasize about sensory deprivation, being blindfolded, gagged, and having my hands immobilized in thick rubber mitts," wrote another.

Would you like to try play piercing? Over-the-knee spanking? Behaving like a brat?

What are the things you *don't* want to try? No breaking the skin? No humiliation play? No resistance? No anal penetration?

What's your safeword? (Remember: tops need safewords, too!)

See Chapter 6, "Communication and Finding Sex Partners," for more on communication skills.

Creating the S/M Scene: Ritual and Theater

Much like a theatrical performance, an S/M scene has characters, a setting, and a beginning, middle, and end. (If you like, you can think of an S/M scene as having much the same framework as a classical three-act play!)

And, like a ritual or spiritual practice, an S/M scene may evoke meaning that's larger than the moment. Shining your Master's boots in the context of a dominance/submission scene will have a far greater meaning than polishing your wingtips alone at home.

What kind of scene do you wish to create? Will your scene involve pain and sensation play? Role-play and costumes? Service? Resistance? Submission?

Who will be the participants? Generally, the top directs the action in the scene and the bottom receives the top's attentions or does the top's wishes. (I say "generally" because you can negotiate these roles to mean anything you wish.) While some women exclusively identity as a top or a bottom, most identify as "switches," alternating between roles. Do you want to be the top? Or the bottom?

What kind of top do you want to be? A slave Master or the Daddy of a disobedient child? Do you wish to inflict pain? Do you want to be obeyed? Worshipped? Resisted? Do you want to "force" yourself on your partner sexually? Do you want to embarrass or humiliate your partner? Do you want to dominate her?

What kind of bottom do you want to be? Do you want to be a slave or a pet? A brat? Do you wish to be controlled? Disciplined? Trained? Punished?

Where will your scene take place? In your bedroom? At a play party? How will your scene start? Many BDSM players use a ritual item, such as a locked collar, as a device for signaling the beginning and end of a scene. At the start of the scene, the collar goes on; at the end of the scene, out comes the key, the lock is snapped open, and the collar goes back in the toy chest.

Pushing the Emotional Edges

Many women opt for play that intentionally pushes their buttons—their psychological buttons, that is. An assault survivor may negotiate a rape scene— as either the victim or the rapist. A survivor of childhood sexual abuse may engage in Daddy/girl or Mommy/boy role play—as either the parent or the child. A woman who struggles with sexual shame may negotiate a scene in which she's "forced" to perform sexually in front of a group of strangers (who, of course, have consented to witness her "humiliation").

> *Thank God this is anonymous. I've never admitted this to anyone, so please protect my privacy. Yes, I fantasize about rape with me being the "victim." This is difficult to express because I've always been such a strong advocate for women's rights. I'm strongly antiviolence and have been in a domestic abuse situation, so I have a difficult time making sense out of my rape fantasy....*

Why would anyone want to do such a thing as enact a rape scenario? Well, often things that make us uncomfortable also arouse us sexually—at times, it seems that the erotic charge is in direct proportion to the degree of unease we feel. Things that make us feel intense shame or anger can also evoke great sexual heat. Playing with emotional hot buttons is, well, hot!

> *I love being taken care of by my Daddy. I have a whole bunch of fantasies where I'm a little girl and am made to please Daddy.*

S/M Is Not Abuse (Abuse Is Not S/M)

S/M play is consensual.	Abuse is not consensual.
S/M is negotiated ahead of time.	Abuse is not negotiated.
S/M has responsible limits and safety rules.	Abuse has no rules or limits and there are no safewords.
S/M is fun, erotic, and loving.	Abuse is manipulative, selfish, and hurtful.
S/M play is enjoyed by both partners.	Abuse victims do not enjoy abuse.
S/M play can be stopped by either partner at any time.	Abuse can't be stopped by the victim/survivor.
S/M players exchange power in agreed upon roles with negotiated boundaries.	Abusers force control using nonconsensual manipulation and violence.
S/M creates a bond of trust.	Abuse destroys trust.

Subjects that we keep under wraps—such as taboo fantasies and imagined complicities—may ignite an especially potent erotic charge. Do you feel guilty about having rape fantasies? Do you feel that your erotic response to your abuse history means you secretly wanted it? Not so! Sex is sex, and abuse is abuse. Sex is consensual, and abuse is not. If you're ever confused about this, compare a negotiated sexual encounter with an incident of abuse. The differences will be quite apparent. See "S/M Is Not Abuse (Abuse Is Not S/M)" above for clarity. In fact, the more you practice negotiation—whether for an S/M scene, a sexual encounter, or a trip to the Grand Canyon with your lover and her two kids—the more easily you'll recognize the difference between the negotiated consensuality of a mutually respectful relationship and the nonnegotiated manipulation and coercion of abuse. Still confused? Try concocting a (non)erotic (non)play list of your abuse history. List everything that happened between you and your abuser. Now, write "yes" next to every item you desired and *explicitly negotiated to achieve*. What? Not writing yet? Of course not! Abuse has nothing in common with consensual sex.

Some women consciously choose to play with the dynamics of abandonment and abuse because they want to understand themselves. Hardly a substitute for a good therapist, yet an S/M partner can help you facilitate a scene in which you get a good look at yourself. What about that traumatic experience is yet unresolved? Where do you feel shame? Where do you feel pride?

You can even turn the story around. S/M can be a tool in healing. As Pat Califia writes, "As a top, I find the old wounds and unappeased hunger. I nourish. I cleanse and close the wounds. I devise and mete out appropriate punishments for old, irrational 'sins.' I trip up the bottom, I see her as she is, and I forgive her and turn her on and make her come, despite her feelings of unworthiness or self-hatred or fear.... A good scene doesn't end with orgasm—it ends with catharsis." [1]

> *My girlfriend surprised me by planning a scene to fulfill my rape fantasy. It was a powerful experience because the concept of rape was twisted and turned into sexual play between two women who trust and care about each other. Being a rape survivor, I thought our rape scene might bring up some old issues, but it actually didn't at all. The scene was totally about us—my girlfriend and me.*

Teach Yourself Some New Tricks

A how-to guide to BDSM could fill volumes (see the "Bibliography"). Here are some favorite techniques, tools, and tricks:

Bondage

Many novice tops discover the pleasure of restraint by tying a partner to the bedpost with their favorite silk scarf. Scarves, twine, and other thin ropes are handy—you probably have some around the house. But they're not the best choice for bondage gear. The knot in that silk scarf will get tighter and tighter with stress and may prove impossible to undo in a hurry. Thin rope or string can cut into the skin like a garrote. Even if the string doesn't pierce the skin, it can cut off the circulation or cause nerve damage.

Thick rope not only is safer, but it's sensual and easy to manipulate. Choose rope that's a minimum of $1/4$ inch thick. A rope that's $1/2$ inch thick will be even more sensuous. Be generous. Get a good long piece—25 to 50 feet. You'll find ropes in a variety of colors, thicknesses, and materials on spools at the hardware store. Good rope isn't cheap—prepare to pay at least 50 cents a foot for high-quality rope.

For those of us whose homes aren't equipped with a St. Andrew's cross—the larger-than-life wooden X that serves as the centerpiece of most dungeons—an ordinary chair will provide a fine bondage station. Seat your partner in the chair and adjust her posture to make sure her back is parallel to the back of the chair, her calves are parallel to the front legs of the chair, and her feet are firmly planted on the floor. Begin by winding rope around her waist, binding her to the chair. If her arms are at her sides, you can include them in the bundle for a mummy-effect. You can leave her breasts free by circling them in a figure eight as you wrap her torso. If her hands are placed in front of her, palms together, you can wind rope in between and around her wrists in a figure eight. And if the back of the chair is low enough, you can bind her hands behind her back; make sure her shoulder joints aren't stressed. Wind rope around each leg, binding it to a leg of the chair.

If you double the rope, you can wind the doubled stand around and around, and then pull the ends through the loop in the middle. You can tie off the job with any easy-to-undo knot; if the knot is out of reach of your partner's hands, she'll be pretty secure.

Since your partner is seated, and her wrists and ankles aren't stressed, too tightly bound, or held in a difficult position, she can stay in this type of bondage comfortably for quite a while.

In some scenes, your goal may be to put the bottom in bondage that allows no movement, leaving her completely at your mercy. In other scenes, the point is to allow the bottom the feel of the ropes themselves. The sensuality of being bound can give her a feeling of being held, much like a corset. As you wind the rope around your partner's torso, tell her that the rope is an extension of you, that it's your desire that's holding her in place. That feeling of being held by her top can provide your partner a delicious feeling of security. Thus bound, she can "let go."

You can even use plastic wrap—rolls and rolls of colored wrap you'll find in the supermarket—to bind your partner to a post, a chair, or a cross. You can wrap her entire torso, save for her pubic area—which you can then attend to with sublime torture! Keep the plastic wrap away from her nose and mouth. To avoid heat prostration, remove the wrappings after 30 minutes or so—depending, of course, on the temperature of the room. On a very hot day, you'd do best to skip the plastic wrap entirely.

Conversely, the most challenging form of bondage for most bottoms is the bondage of will—no bindings, no rope, no lock and key. Simple obedience to a top's command—"Stand there and don't move!"—will stretch her capacity for submission. It's especially difficult to take a whipping or caning when held in place only by one's own desire to submit.

Restraints

Wrist and ankle restraints are often the first bondage gear we buy outside of a hardware store. You can buy fairly inexpensive wrist restraints made of cloth webbing and Velcro, or you can go upscale with beautifully crafted leather restraints. What's important is that the material be wide enough to avoid stress on the joints and that the restraints fit snugly and close securely—many are designed for use with padlocks. They all feature a ring through which you can loop rope or attach a chain. Many women prefer handcuffs—which evoke fantasies of law enforcement officers capturing escaped prisoners. If you're going to use handcuffs, buy a quality pair designed with a safety stop to lock them in at a comfortable point. Cheaper handcuffs tend to get tighter and tighter with stress. Don't lose the key!

A few basic rules for wrist and angle restraint: If restraints are too tight, blood circulation will be restricted. Check your partner's fingers and feet for numbness. Don't keep her hands above her head for longer than 30 minutes—she could faint. Don't allow your partner's weight to place stress on joints—wrist and angle restraints aren't suitable for suspension bondage.

Sensory Deprivation

Depriving someone of her senses creates mystery. With her eyes covered by a blindfold, your partner will listen to every creak and rustle to figure out where you are and what you're doing. Since she doesn't know whether you're picking out a soft deerskin flogger or a stinging cane, she can't anticipate the sensation...which will be more intense for being such a surprise. (Keep that in mind as you get ready to whack her with that toy—a little will go a long way with a blindfolded partner.)

A gag will disable your partner's ability to communicate with words or even sound. Not being able to speak may make her feel especially helpless. Remember, of course, that in negotiating use of a gag, you must arrange a visual safeword. Will your partner be able to snap her fingers? Hold up one thumb? You must also make sure that the device you use as a gag will permit your partner to breathe easily and to swallow saliva without choking.

A hood combines the effects of a blindfold with a sense of being enveloped. A spandex body bag will extend that feeling to the entire body. Some women find the experience of wearing a hood and body bag very securing and even transcendent—alone in the dark with only your own internal awareness, your experience of yourself is greatly heightened. Yet some people find hoods and body bags terrifying. If you use one, make sure the hood is well ventilated. Again, don't forget to arrange for an appropriate method of communicating a safeword.

You can make a hood from cut-up pantyhose. Tie a scarf or blindfold around your partner's eyes and then slip the thigh of the pantyhose over her head. Double it over to make it thicker.

Spanking

Often the first kind of erotic beating many women try is a good (or "bad") spanking. Spanking can be very erotic because the hand comes in direct contact with the buttocks. The heat and force of the hand sends ripples of sensation throughout the pelvic area. With the bottom's pelvis firmly planted on the top's lap, the clitoris can grind against the knee with each downward stroke of the hand.

A spanking can feel very sensual, with gentle pats and caresses, or punishing, with hard-pounding strikes of the palm against flesh. A spanking can leave very personal marks—the outline of a hand on a loved one's ass.

Many women have strong emotional associations with spanking, as they may have been spanked as a child—many women have similarly strong associations with face slapping. "There is something very personal about being hit with an open hand," wrote one woman. "It accentuates the power dynamic."

Paddling

A paddle is an easy tool to wield for a novice top. Paddles are easy to find and require less skill than other implements. You can buy fur-covered paddles, or paddles with fur on one side and leather on the other. You can find a hard wooden paddle, like the ones fraternity members use. You can even use a Ping Pong paddle. Strike only the fleshy parts of the buttocks and upper thighs. Don't strike bone or joints. Find the "sweet" spot of the ass—that place where the upper thighs meet the buttocks.

Caning

Canes are thin rods made of rattan, plastic, or Fiberglas. Many people are utterly terrified of canes—and with good reason! Canes can produce a menacing amount of pain and leave welts. A formal British caning lays "six of the best" in a mean row along the thighs and buttocks. The red lines sting in a particularly nasty way. Good caning skill takes practice.

Yet because canes are so scary, they're effective in producing an emotional reaction as well as a physical one. Many bottoms who at first reluctantly bend over for the cane eventually admit that they love getting caned.

Whipping

Whips are sensuous and beautiful…and require a degree of skill. Whips are harder to control than your hand, a paddle, or a cane. There are many different kinds of whips, such as floggers, cat o' nine tails, quirts, and signal whips, to name a few.

Floggers are multi-tailed whips. A flogger can be constructed from a variety of materials, including deerskin, cowhide, bull hide, elk and buffalo skin—or even heavy rubber. A flogging can be sensual and subtle or pounding, and a good, hard flogging can feel like deep tissue massage. Cat o' nine tails are just what they sound like—floggers made of nine braided strands. They have the weight of a flogger, but the individual braided strands can do more damage than the individual strands of a flogger. Single-tailed whips, like 4-foot signal whips used to drive working dogs, require considerable skill to use safely.

Janette Heartwood, a well-respected whipmaker, identifies three aspects of whipping: accuracy, intensity, and connection.[2] Accuracy and intensity, she says, are "manual skills" that you can develop by practicing on inanimate objects, such as a pillow, a stuffed animal, or a padded leather bar stool.

Accuracy is the ability to control a whip so that when the tails fly through the air, the tips land where you've chosen. "A whip should be visualized as an extension of your arm," she says. Floggers and cat o' nine tails will wrap around the hip if you're not careful in your aim. Since the ends of the whip are moving at a higher rate of speed than the midsection, your worst damage will be done where you least want it—the hip bone and the soft flesh of the lower belly. Practice with a pillow until you're sure that you can aim the ends of the whip in exactly the spot you have selected—for instance, the upper back or the fleshiest part of the buttocks.

Do not whip joints. Do not whip areas of the body where bones lack protection of fleshy padding—such as the tailbone, spine and ribs. Do not whip the abdomen or kidneys. Keep the tails of the whip away from the face. You can whip the breasts and vulva *lightly*.

Heartwood defines *intensity* is the "severity" of sensation and the "cadence" with which it's delivered.

How much of the flogger makes contact with the flesh will determine how thuddy or stingy the sensation. If you get really good, you can send the ends of the whip whizzing by so that they barely brush the skin. That will result in a very stingy sensation. A dead-on whump of the heaviest part of the flogger will result in a heavy, thuddy sensation that many women find really satisfying, like a good hard deep-muscle massage.

Connection, says Heartwood, is the "ethereal" aspect of the scene that draws on the top's "empathy, centeredness, and creativity." Connection is the ability to deliver a whipping that fulfills the needs of both the top *and* the bottom.

After a good, hard whipping, you can send your partner into orbit by lightly running your fingernails along her skin. The contrast will send her into fits of giggles as she begs you to stop. ("Stop! Don't stop! *Stop!*")

Hanky Code

Do you flag left or right? A hanky worn in the left-rear pocket identifies you as a top; a hanky worn in the right-rear pocket identifies you as a bottom. Hanky codes have a long history in the gay men's community; like slang, the hanky code has evolved from generation to generation and from community to community. When it comes to sex, most hanky codes assume the top is the insertive partner and the bottom is the receptive one—but, of course, that's a matter of negotiation!

Worn on the Left	Color	Worn on the Right
Heavy S/M top	Black	Heavy S/M bottom
Latex fetish top	Charcoal	Latex fetish bottom
Bondage top	Gray	Bondage bottom
Anal sex top	Dark blue	Anal sex bottom
Oral sex top	Light blue	Oral sex bottom
Light S/M top	Robin's-egg blue	Light S/M bottom
Seeks menstruating partners	Maroon	Menstruating
Fist-fucking top	Red	Fist-fucking bottom
Shaving top	Red/white stripe	Shaving bottom
Tit torture top	Dark pink	Tit torture bottom
Strap-on top	Light pink	Strap-on bottom
"Anything goes" top	Orange	"Anything goes" bottom
Golden showers top	Yellow	Golden showers bottom
Piercing top	Purple	Piercing bottom
Likes drag queens	Lavender	Drag queen
Daddy	Hunter green	Seeks a Daddy
Uniform top	Olive drab	Uniform bottom
Spanking top	Fuchsia	Spanking bottom
Scat top	Brown	Scat bottom
Rimming top	Beige	Rimming bottom
Seeks novices	White	Novice
Victorian scene top	White lace	Victorian scene bottom
Voyeur	White velvet	Exhibitionist

You can economize in many areas of your toy chest, but if you're going to invest in a whip, select one from a whipmaker whose creations are respected among experienced S/M players. See the "Resources" for suggestions.

Clamps

You restrict blood flow when you use clamps. They hurt when they go on, and hurt more when they come off, as the blood rushes back into the area that was constricted. You can experiment on yourself. Try attaching clothespins or small clips to the inside of your arm, sides of your breasts, or nipples.

You can purchase several different types of nipple clamps (which can double as labia clamps): tweezer-style clamps, alligator clamps with teeth (often rubber-covered), and Japanese clover-shaped clamps that get tighter when pulled. Clamps come in pairs linked by a thin chain. You can hang 1-ounce weights from the chain. Don't keep clamps on for more than 20 to 30 minutes, since restricting blood flow can damage tissue and nerves.

A zipper is an extremely nasty (or nice) toy made by stringing together ordinary wooden clothespins. Slide a piece of string through the metal hole in the center of the clothespin and tie knots on either side so that the clothespin can't slide along the string. Repeat at 2-inch intervals until you have a dozen clothespins evenly spaced on the string. Attach the zipper by applying each clothespin to your partner's upper arms, thighs, or torso, and leave them on for about ten minutes. Then yank the string to "pull the zipper." Yowza.

Sensation Play

You can manipulate sensation in all sorts of clever ways. Two popular methods are to play with texture (feathers and fur mitts alternating with fingernails or neuro wheels) and temperature (Tiger's Balm or hot wax alternating with ice cubes).

Common household candles are fine for wax play—in fact they're preferred over beeswax, which melts at a much higher temperature. With your partner lying on her back, hold a lit candle several feet above her torso. Tilt the candle so that the hot wax drips down on her chest one drop at a time. The wax will sear as it meets her skin. The burning sensation will fade to a pleasant glow after a moment. You can intensify the sensation by holding the candle closer to her body.

What goes on must come off! You have to get all that melted wax off her skin, which can itself be fun. You can carefully pick individual bits of wax off her skin with the tip of a knife. The sensation of the knife barely scratching her skin as the pieces of wax are peeled away can be very intense on her already-sensitive flesh.

Keep hot wax away from the face and genitals, and keep flames away from bed sheets!

Play Piercings

Many women are devoted to blood play, which may include temporary piercing with sterile needles and knife play with or without breaking the skin. Any opening of the skin opens a channel to the emotions as well. It's important to respect the potential for vulnerability in blood play, as well as to respect the need for sterile procedures. *These are advanced S/M techniques. Do not attempt play piercings or cuttings without instruction from an experienced player.*

Many women enjoy the intensity and intimacy of temporary piercings. In play piercing, sterile hypodermic needles (ranging from 25 gauge to 16 gauge) are inserted under a layer of skin so thin that you may be able to see the needle through the skin's surface. (Never poke a needle into the flesh; slide it gently under the topmost layer of skin.)

You can pierce any fleshy area of the body, such as the breasts, chest, or upper arms. Unless you're a very experienced piercer, avoid areas dense with nerves, such as the face. In addition to sterile needles, you'll need latex gloves, alcohol wipes, and a proper container for disposing of used sharps.

Remember that any time the skin is opened, there's a possibility of infection. Clean the area with alcohol and wear gloves. Be careful not to stick yourself with a used needle. Don't reuse needles. Dispose of needles properly.

You'll find step-by-step instructions for play piercing in the Web links below, as well as information on obtaining needles. Do *not* attempt blood play without proper instruction.

"Home Despot"

You can create a dungeon at home with a little ingenuity—plus a trip to your local hardware store. (You'll never look at the store the same—and the folks in the logo aprons probably won't look at you the same either.)

You can attach eyebolts to the ceiling, the frame of a doorway, or other solid surface. Make sure you find a stud or crossbeam; the bolt will tear through plaster or Sheetrock the first time you play with a feisty bottom! You can attach lengths of chain to the eyebolts using panic snaps, and then secure the chain to wrist and ankle restraints. Panic snaps are clips designed to release easily—even with a person weighing them down. You'll find spools of chain of all gauges and colors at a good hardware store. Examine the links carefully; avoid chain that has sharp points where the links close. Generally, a heavier chain will be safer to use (it can't cut into a partner's skin), has smoother links, and will produce a much scarier effect! (Try blindfolding your partner before you attach her to the chains; let her listen to the chain clanking.)

While you're browsing for chain and eyebolts, check out the displays of rope, shackles, clips, clothespins, kitchen utensils, candles, and first aid and safety supplies.

You can buy or make a sling, which you can hang from hooks in the ceiling or from a frame. See the "Resources" for vendors of S/M gear.

Make sure the room you intend to use as your dungeon has adequate lighting and is clean—particularly if you plan to engage in play piercing. You can install soundproofing insulation if you're worried about neighbors—or invest in a gag!

How Do You Know What You Want?

"Mostly, what I want to know is how do you know what you would like if you've never done it?" wrote one woman who expressed a fascination with BDSM—but little actual experience. "How do you know whether to ask for a Fiberglas cane, say, or a riding crop? Obviously, my perverted bottom child-self has had many fantasies about being hit—but I don't know that I pictured precisely with what. So, does one just say, 'I'll let you know if I don't like it'?"

Faced with an endless list of possibilities, how do you know what you'll like? Or what you even want to try? Here are some suggestions:

- *Begin with fantasy.* What produces the most heat for you? What do you imagine when you close your eyes? "I fantasize having my hands bound—not so that I will be hurt, but so that I can't touch my lover. I love feeling desired and knowing that everything she does, she does completely of her own free will."

- *Experiment with sensations on yourself.* From wooden spoons to clothespins, you've probably got an arsenal of implements of torture in your home.

- *Go shopping.* You can visit a leather S/M store and handle the toys. Which ones feel good in your hands? Or turn you on right there in the aisle? You can shop online as well. While you won't get a tactile sense of the potential of various toys, you'll get some impressive visuals. Some web sites selling S/M gear show beautifully designed whips, crops, hoods, and other bondage devices.

- *Experiment with a friend*—outside of any scene or sexual context. Take turns paddling each other with that wooden spoon or swinging a belt against bare flesh.

- *Negotiate a scene.* Many experienced tops enjoy playing with novice bottoms. Why? It makes S/M new for them, too. Tops who play with novice bottoms have all sorts of tricks for helping their partners discover what works best for them. One popular method is to "calibrate" the bottom to each type of sensation. The top asks the bottom to assign each sensation a value on a 1-to-10 scale, with 1 being hardly perceptible and 10 being unbearable to the point of calling a safeword. The top then treats the bottom to a feast of sensations, from the lightest caress of a soft deerskin flogger to the most unforgiving whack of a wooden paddle. In this way, the bottom can discover what she likes in a very safe context. The top can discover how the bottom responds to the top's particular style and decide whether she might want to explore further play.

"But won't it be embarrassing to say my safeword? Won't I look like a wuss if I can't take it?" Not at all! Taking a lot of pain doesn't make you a better bottom, nor does being able to push a partner to scarier edges make you a better top. Experienced players use their safewords all the time. Your ability to say your safeword as needed is what makes you a good bottom and a safe player. Likewise, a top's ability to respond to your safeword is what makes her a safe partner.

"But I want to be a top. Isn't a novice top a little, well, unconvincing?" Hardly! What makes you want to exert control over another person? When did you discover your desire to inflict pain? That urge to dominate is real; don't doubt yourself. Many novice tops play with notice bottoms, discovering together their likes and dislikes. Others play with experienced players who are willing to teach from the bottom, so to speak. You may wish to enter into a mentoring relationship with an experienced top. See the "Resources" to find a BDSM-oriented e-mail discussion list or a local S/M organization.

Toys for BDSM Play

In your BDSM play you can use toys ranging from homemade and appropriated items (see "Home Despot," above) to beautifully handcrafted leather and wooden implements. You can choose from whips, canes, crops, bondage furniture, hoods, restraints, and many, many other items. It's not unusual for a well-equipped dungeon to boast thousands of dollars worth of toys and other devices.

So how can an ordinary girl play on a budget? For starters, check the "Resources" for mail-order companies that offer inexpensive BDSM toys. Then, make some choices. Which toys must you have in your collection? Which can you improvise? Or borrow before you buy?

Canes and riding crops are relatively inexpensive. Impact toys like paddles and straps can be easily improvised with common household items. Of course, if you're talented, you can learn to make your own toys.

That Sounds Dangerous!

Yes, there *is* danger in S/M play. You can't restrict movement or stress the body without some risk. And if you also administer punishment, make demands for

A Novice's Story

My friend had just ended her relationship with her girlfriend, who was the only top she'd ever played with. She'd never participated in her local S/M community. She'd never played with anyone other than her ex-girlfriend and she was at a loss as to where to find partners.

So, she attended a workshop on negotiation at a local erotic boutique taught by a well-known professional dominatrix. Emboldened by her new negotiation skills, she approached the teacher after the workshop and asked her if she ever worked with women clients. Mistress was more than pleased by the idea of working with a woman client and offered my friend a reduced fee.

The Mistress offered a sliding scale of from $150 to $250 for a two- to three-hour scene, plus a 45-minute phone conversation in which they negotiated the scene. (A session with a professional dominatrix is not prostitution—since it does not involved the exchange of sex for money. "Sex" is usually defined as involving some form of direct genital contact.)

The day after the session, my friend was dancing in her seat at the café where we met for coffee. Her eyes sparkled with excitement and her face glowed. Soon after we sat down, she asked if I wanted to see the marks from her play piercing and before I could say *Story of O* she had pulled down the neckline of her jersey to reveal the little two red dots where the needle had entered and then exited her chest.

My friend was three times a virgin: she had never been naked in front of a stranger (in an erotic context), she had never negotiated a "real" scene, and she had never paid for an erotic encounter.

As I admired her marks, she chattered on, telling me of the Mistress's private dungeon, the whole wall just of multicolored and textured whips, and the rack to which she had been bound. Images and snippets of memory came tumbling out—the Mistress commanding her to select one whip she would like and one that frightened her; the elaborate rope bondage embracing her thighs, arms, and torso; the mixture of devotion and arousal the Mistress stirred in her; the tears that came finally as she released the grief over the loss of her lover/top. "At some point during the whipping, she let me suck her hand—and I was gone."

---

extreme levels of obedience and patience, concoct humiliating or embarrassing scenarios, or otherwise toy with a person's emotional resilience, you're playing the edge indeed.

Good players are safety conscious. They stand by the motto "Safe, sane, consensual." Safety is supported by the use of safewords to stop play when necessary, sanity by the practice of playing when emotionally present (and not playing when inebriated or high), and consent by the practice of negotiation.

Any S/M top worth her leathers can tell you how to restrain your partner without restricting blood flow or causing nerve damage; precisely where on the human body you can and can't safely aim your whip or paddle; and what emergency items to pack in your toy bag.

That same top can also tell you about emotional care—the importance of showering your partner with praise and tenderness, supporting her desires, nurturing her abilities, and respecting her limits.

Yet S/M is not without risks. Physical accidents, unintended emotional harm, and the residue of intense vulnerability can leave either partner hurting. S/M players are dedicated to the play in spite of the risks.

BDSM Play—Safely

A guide to BDSM safety could fill the pages of this entire chapter. The bottom line is this: Do not pretend to expertise you do not have. *If you don't know how, don't do it!*

Here are some safety pointers: Make sure all your devices work and are of good enough quality to be safe. Never leave a person in bondage unattended. Watch for tingling in hands and feet or stress on joints. Use panic snaps so that you can release your partner quickly; release the feet before the arms so that she doesn't fall over. Keep bandage scissors on hand to cut through rope. Keep keys to handcuffs, restraints, and collars in your pocket.

Do not whip bones or joints—see "Whipping," above.

Never play when under the influence of alcohol or drugs. Certainly, don't take any medication that dulls the senses.

Provide for your partner's aftercare. Make sure juice or a high-protein snack is available. After an intense scene, the bottom may be shaky. Make sure she's kept warm. Don't leave her unattended.

Create safety by playing at a party before playing privately. Dungeon monitors and other experienced players can help you learn how to do things safely.

Community adds yet another level of safety to S/M play. In a community, we're all accountable. BDSM players are known to their peers. You can find out if the people you admire consider that potential partner a safe, responsible player—*before* she's got you trussed up to her bedposts!

Where to Learn More

S/M and leather communities have a long tradition of mentoring novices. Many experienced S/M players love to pass on their knowledge. BDSM organizations, such as those listed in the "Resources," are great places to learn how to use a flogger, what you can do with hot wax, or the finer points of negotiation. You can watch demos of activities you may not even want to try—yet! Often workshops and educational events are open to nonmembers.

You'll find a number of guides in the "Bibliography" that offer detailed information on techniques for BDSM play.

Suggested Web Links:

AltSex Pages
    www.altsex.org
The soc.subculture.bondage-bdsm FAQ List
    www.unrealities.com/adult/ssbb/faq.htm
Play Piercing
    www.sexuality.org/l/bdsm/needle.html

Notes
  1. Pat Califia, *Public Sex: The Culture of Radical Sex* (Cleis Press, 1994), 163.
  2. Janette Heartwood, Heartwood Whips of Passion, web site, www.heartwoodwhips.com

Source of Sidebar
"S/M Is Not Abuse (Abuse Is Not S/M)" is reprinted with permission from a pamphlet published by AABL (see "Resources").

chapter fourteen

Play Parties
and Public Sex

*I really like to have public sex. It's the whole idea of doing something naughty
and the possibility of getting caught.*

MANY LESBIANS AND BISEXUAL WOMEN LOVE SEX IN PUBLIC. Does that mean they have sex in the back seats of cars, public bathrooms, or the park? Well, they might—though such scenarios carry serious risks, including the risk of assault or arrest.

Public sex needn't be dangerous or illegal—nor must you involve bystanders as unwilling voyeurs to your scene. Celebrating sex in public doesn't necessarily mean that you get down with your girlfriend under the pool table at your local lesbian bar. Public sex can include many safe, consensual forms of sexual expression that you can enjoy outside the privacy of your bedroom—from attendance at an erotic performance to a night of group sex at a play party.

Commercial Sex

Most people think of prostitution—the exchange of sex for money—when they think of commercial sex. Yet commercial sex can include any form of sexual expression or entertainment that you pay to enjoy—from the purchase of erotic books, magazines, and videos to the dollar you slip into the lacy thong of a dancer at a strip club.

Prostitution is illegal in most of the United States and many other countries. Generally "prostitution" is defined as exchanging sex for money; and usually "sex" is defined as involving some form of direct genital contact. So, in many places where prostitution is illegal, it may be perfectly permissible to charge clients for private sessions with a dominatrix or to host erotic performances and sex parties. Of course, local laws, regulations, and enforcement practices vary widely.

We usually don't think of women as consumers of commercial sex. Yet any dyke who has attended an all-women strip show, purchased a copy of *On Our Backs* or *Best Lesbian Erotica*, rented a lesbian sex video, called a phone sex line, logged onto a cybersex site, or bought a ticket to an explicitly erotic performance has paid for sexual entertainment.

Of course, it's an open secret that many lesbians and bisexual women work in the sex industry. The ubiquitous girl–girl sex scenes found in porn videos marketed to heterosexual men are often performed by bisexual or lesbian women passing as heterosexual women pretending to be lesbians! Lesbians and bisexual women who work in the sex industry are often delighted to find women in their audiences and among their clientele.

Other lesbians—whether paid or not—strip for the pleasure of seducing a room full of women.

> *I frequently work as a dyke stripper at a local dyke cabaret night. The first time I stripped I had forgotten that folks would be tucking money into my underwear. I'd never even seen a stripper before—and here I was doing a favor for a friend. The audience was so supportive! I felt so sexy! Folks were whispering dirty things in my ears as they tucked bills into my g-string. I felt like the sex goddess of the universe. I've never stripped for men, and I don't think I want to. But for women it's so sexy!*

Unless you frequent lesbian strip shows or sex parties, you may have never observed other lesbians having sex—live and in the flesh. Lesbian-produced videos and magazines offer the opportunity to see images of real dykes having real sex. You can't pop a low-budget, lesbian-made video into the VCR and miss the fact that these are real lesbians having real sex for the pleasure of putting their lust on exhibition—something women just aren't supposed to do!

For many women, cybersex is their first experience with actually having public sex—rather than viewing it. You can enter an unmoderated chat room, "listen" in until you feel comfortable, and then jump into the fray. Cybersex offers a safe introduction to anonymous sex, since you can "pick up" another woman, "go private" by creating a private chat room for your encounter, and have cybersex—without risk of STDs or unwanted entanglements.

What about live sex? Where can a lesbian or bisexual woman go to enjoy live sexual performances? Some women go to strip clubs. You can go in a group, cheer on the erotic dancers, and even pay for a lap dance.

Play Parties

I had the most intense orgasm of my life while being caressed, kissed, and penetrated by two women. This was just about the best sex I have ever experienced!

A play party is a gathering where people engage in sex. There are all types of play parties—some are for women only and others are "pansexual," welcoming all genders, all sexual styles, and all sexual orientations.

Some parties are small, private affairs—a lesbian invites three friends over for a romp in her bed. Others are large public events, hosting as many as 200 women who have learned of the event from a flier or ad. Most play parties are semipublic. The host draws up an invitation list, encouraging guests to bring their friends, who are then added to the list for future events. Most party hosts charge a fee to cover space rental, safer-sex supplies, food, and other expenses.

Parties, of course, come in all flavors, with styles as individual as their hosts. From sensual affairs with hot tubs and scrumptious buffets to dungeon parties where women engage in elaborately negotiated BDSM scenes, you'll find play parties to suit a wide range of tastes. Some parties begin with games and icebreakers; others feature rituals intended to create a particular mood.

12 Reasons to Go to a Sex Party

1. You can nurture your inner exhibitionist. You can perform for an audience of eager voyeurs.

2. You can indulge in sensory overload, watching and hearing others engage in sexual activities—while you're having sex!

3. You can leave your inhibitions at the door and try sexual activities you've only imagined. Nothing like a change of venue to make you feel adventurous.

4. Your body image will get a big boost when you see women of all shapes and sizes being admired erotically.

5. You can scream out your pleasure (or pain) without worrying about your neighbors.

6. You'll get plenty of encouragement for being a slut. You may even get a round of applause when you come!

7. You can make friends and find sex partners.

8. You can have group sex, and you can have sex with strangers in a safe environment.

9. You can play on good equipment—like a St. Andrew's cross or sling. You can play with that new 6-foot single-tailed whip you can't safely swing in your living room!

10. You can enact your favorite public sex fantasy without the risk of encountering cops and queer-bashers.

11. You can have sex without the complications of dating and romance, or waking up with a U-Haul parked on your front lawn.

12. You can spice up your marriage. Even if you and your partner wish to have sex only with each other, you can enjoy an entirely new erotic environment.

What does a play party look like? Typically, you'll find a social area with refreshments, an area to change out of street clothes and into fetish wear, and a play area. Some party spaces even have showers. You may find an impressive array of dungeon equipment, including St. Andrew's crosses, racks, cages, and slings. You may even find a gynecologist's examination table! Or, you may find a room lined with futons or foam mattresses.

You'll see women naked, or wearing all manner of fetish gear, including corsets, g-strings, dildos and harnesses, chaps, and stiletto heels. You'll find women watching others having sex, or chatting in small groups, as at any other party. You may see couples in discreet corners, lost in deep kisses; a group of women in a "puppy pile" of jumbled limbs and torsos; or a daisy chain of women engaging in oral sex. You may see women getting fisted in slings. You'll certainly get to see and hear many women's orgasms!

At a BDSM party, you'll find women tied to whipping posts, crosses, bondage tables, racks, and (in standing bondage) to eyebolts in a low ceiling. You'll hear the crack of single-tailed whips, the smack of paddles on buttocks, and, of course, lots of sighs and screams!

You'll see women practicing safer sex, too. You can learn how to introduce latex and other barriers into a scene. You may see a woman erotically teasing her partner as she slowly slips on a glove or licking a partner's thighs as she spreads a dental dam over her vulva. You'll see women lube up condom-covered dildos and butt plugs, and slip gloves over the heads of electric vibrators.

Many party hosts post safer-sex rules. They may be as simple as "no exchange of bodily fluid" or quite detailed, specifying when gloves and condoms are to be used. You may find etiquette rules posted as well. Hosts may remind guests to ask before touching and to refrain from interrupting others' play. Often S/M parties employ dungeon monitors who can help guests with safety concerns. In many communities, "safeword" has itself become the universal safeword—if you call out "safeword," folks will come running!

How to Have Fun at a Sex Party

How can you have a good time at a sex party? Lower your expectations. If your goal for the evening is to have sex with a particular individual or to meet the woman of your dreams, you may go home disappointed. Set a reasonable goal for yourself. For instance, just showing up and watching a scene, or saying hello to one person you don't know, is a reasonable objective for a first play party.

Play parties can be great places to learn how the principles of negotiation and safer sex work in "real" life. In your everyday life, you might feel awkward asking for sex or turning down an offer of a date. Being surrounded by women who boldly state their erotic interests and preferences gives you support for asking for what *you* want, too. You can practice saying, "Would you like to…" and "I'd love to…" and "No, thanks" in an erotic context.

Give yourself permission to seek out any form of pleasure that feels right to you. You can get a foot rub. You can be fed strawberries as you watch women engage in sex. You can try new sexual activities, experiment with roles and costumes, and have sex with six women—if you find willing participants and have the stamina! You can play with women or men, or both, if you so desire.

Don't do anything that doesn't feel right to you. Attendance at a pansexual party doesn't necessarily mean you're interested in having sex with men—regardless of whether you identify as lesbian or bisexual. In fact, going to a play party doesn't obligate you to have sex at all! You may be wholeheartedly appreciated as an enthusiastic voyeur.

Don't want to go to a party alone? So take a friend or lover—just be sure you discuss your expectations for the evening *before* you get to the party. Will you be having sex with each other? With others as well? Is it OK if one of you goes off on her own to engage in sex play? Can the other watch? What happens if one of you wants to leave?

What if you see a scene so erotically compelling you just *have* to join in? Can you join a group engaged in sex? You can make your presence known *subtly* without interrupting or crowding the scene. Wait until you have an opportunity to make eye contact. Smile. Let the women involved in the scene initiate communication. If there's no interest, move on. If there is, ask: "May I join you?"

Where to Find Play Parties

You may have to hunt to find a play party if you don't live in a big city—or if you're new in town. Your local S/M organization or sex-toy boutique is the best place to start when looking for sex parties. If that doesn't work, get online and ask members of your favorite sexually oriented e-mail discussion list if they know of any parties in your area. See the "Resources" for suggestions.

Play Party Etiquette

Don't...

- Don't touch anyone without asking permission.
- Don't crowd scenes. If someone asks you to back off, do so graciously.
- Don't try to join a scene unless invited.
- Don't interrupt someone's scene or play or talk loudly in the play area.
- Don't gape judgmentally. Don't snicker.
- Don't borrow toys without asking.

Do...

- Respect the party rules regarding safer sex—even if you and your date are fluid-bonded. Why? You'll set a good example and encourage others to practice safe sex.
- Clean up after yourself. Wipe down surfaces. Pick up your used gloves and condoms and dispose of them properly.
- Be generous with your compliments.
- Bring food if the invitation requests it. Real food—homemade bread, veggies and dip, and organic juices—will be appreciated by tired souls at 3 A.M.
- Respect the anonymity of your fellow party-goers. Your erotic tales will be just as spectacular without names or identifying details.
- Thank your host. Giving a sex party is a big risk!

How to Throw a Safer-Sex Party

You can host an erotic event of your own. Be forewarned that hosting a play party will require more work than you probably can anticipate and will stretch your sexual self-confidence—you really *are* putting your desires out there when you host an explicitly sexual event.

What kind of party would you host? An intimate evening of group sex? An S/M play party? An erotic cabaret with strippers, dancing, food, and sex? (You could even organize your event as a fundraiser and raffle off sex toys and erotic videos.)

Are sex clubs legal? Will you get arrested for hosting a private play party? A public play party? Is it legal to charge admission for the event? Can you advertise?

Laws regulating sex businesses vary from city to city and country to country. In some cities, nudity isn't legal in an establishment that serves alcohol. In other cities, sex clubs are legal if the patrons purchase memberships. In many places, no such business would be tolerated at all. You can ask the proprietor of a local sex club or gay bathhouse or your local civil liberties organization for information on regulations in your area.

Whom would you like to invite? Will you limit the party to close friends and lovers? Or will you send an invitation to every known lesbian within a 30-mile radius? Talk to your friends as you plan your party. What kind of event would *they* enjoy?

Your invitation can reassure your friends that participating in erotic play is entirely voluntary. Encourage them to bring their favorite food, beverages, and music—people often feel more comfortable at an event if they have a role to play. You can also invite your most gregarious (and least-threatening) friends to take shifts at the door.

Don't forget to remind your guests not to wear scented cosmetics or perfumes if any of your guests may be chemically sensitive. Also let your guests know what kinds of safer-sex supplies you'll provide. Will you have Lollyes dams? Plastic wrap? Latex gloves? Water-based lube? Will you have latex alternatives, like nitrile gloves and polyurethane condoms? Glycerin-free lube? If not, say so—let your guests know that they need to bring these supplies.

Will your space be accessible to disabled guests? Say so on the invitation, and be specific. Don't say "wheelchair accessible" if there are three steps up to your front door or if your bathroom door isn't large enough to accommodate a wheelchair. State whether or not your event will be ASL interpreted. What other accessibility issues might you address in your event planning? Here's a prime opportunity to consult with disabled lesbians and bisexual women in your community. Ask what would make the event feasible for them.

Where will the party be held? Will it be big enough to accommodate your guest list? Is there parking? Public transportation? Make sure the space is adequately heated (or cooled, depending on the season) and *clean*. (Nothing worse than grabbing a sticky lube bottle to find it's coated with dust!) Will you

Carol Queen on Voyeurs and Exhibitionists

Voyeurs who bring love and appreciation to their watching are another species altogether. In a sense, everyone in a public sex environment is both voyeur and exhibitionist—if not, they'd probably prefer to stay home. But dyed-in-the-wool voyeurs are the glue that helps a party cohere. They add sexual energy instead of taking it away; their rapt and watchful presence can turn up the heat on any scene.

If voyeurs add glue, exhibitionists add kindling. Many times, my partner and I have fueled a sluggish, slow-to-start party by placing ourselves in the center of the room and beginning to do something explicit or outrageous. First we attract the voyeurs. The next thing we know, couples and groups have formed all around us. The party has ignited.

---

borrow BDSM equipment? Futons? Cover mattresses and other upholstered surfaces with plastic sheets and then with cloth sheets. Make sure you provide plenty of paper towels and trash receptacles.

You can employ a few tricks to get things rolling. You can "seed" your guest list with a few exhibitionist friends whom you can count on to ignite the rest of the crowd, as Carol Queen suggests above. You can start the evening with a ritual, erotic performance, or a game, such as passing sex toys around a circle—hands free.

Soon you won't have to worry about stoking the action—even your most introverted guests will be happily occupied. And you'll be so busy restocking lube and safer-sex supplies that you'll hardly have a minute to wonder what's become of all those shy friends who swore they'd be too nervous to "do" anything!

Suggested Web Links:

ALT.SEX.BONDAGE FAQ

    www.altsex.org/altsex-home.html

SOCIETY FOR HUMAN SEXUALITY

    Enjoying and Hosting Erotic Events

    www.sexuality.org/ehee.html

CRAVE

    Music for BDSM parties, featuring classical, New Age, goth, and techno selections, as well as erotica and information on BDSM from a lesbian submissive's viewpoint.

    www.webmistress.org

SOURCE OF SIDEBAR
Carol Queen, *Real Live Nude Girl: Chronicles of Sex-Positive Culture* (Cleis Press, 1997).

chapter fifteen

Sex Toys and Accoutrements

My silicone dildo has wonderful ridges that rub my G-spot just the right way. If I was stuck on a deserted island, this is the one sex toy I would take with me.

NOT LONG AGO, THERE WERE FEW PLACES TO BUY SEX TOYS other than porn shops catering primarily to men. In those days, sex toys were hardly designed with lesbians in mind. Marketed as novelty items, many toys were quite shoddy. Along with silly floppy dildos, you could find battery-operated vibrators so cheaply made they'd land in the trash quicker than you could say "preorgasmic." Of course, classic porn shops are still around, and while you may get a kick out of the corny displays of toys in lurid packaging, many women find these shops truly awful.

Along came Good Vibrations in 1977. Clean, friendly, staffed mostly by women, Good Vibrations set out to promote the philosophy "sexual pleasure is everyone's birthright."[1]

Not only did Good Vibrations spawn a host of other lesbian-friendly sex stores throughout North America, it also proved to be fertile ground for the creative juices of "sexperts" like Susie Bright who got their sex education selling dildos and vibrators there. Now you'll find dozens of retail and mail-order sources for well-made, attractive dildos, vibrators, harnesses, and other toys designed with you in mind. You can get accurate information and helpful advice, along with books, magazines, videos, toys, fetish gear, and safer-sex supplies.

Introducing Sex Toys into Partner Play

The same communications skills you use to negotiate any type of sex will help you introduce your partner to your favorite sex toys. See "Sex Talk Guidelines" in Chapter 6, "Communication and Finding Sex Partners."

- *Tell your partner your sex-toy fantasies.* She may have no idea what you want to do with that vibrating cock ring.

- *Bring up the subject in a relaxed setting.*

- *Speak in positives.* She may jump to the conclusion that if you want to bring your vibrator to bed you must find her techniques inadequate. Tell her what you like about her sexual style *and* what you like about sex toys.

- *Trust your senses.* Are you concerned that sex toys are contrived or unnatural? One woman wrote, "I used to believe that 'real' lesbians only had sex in a 'natural' way—hands, mouth, tongue, fist." The blood pulsing through your clitoris, the contractions of your vaginal and anal muscles, the rush of pleasure through your genitals—all are deliciously "natural"! So trust your body, not your judgments.

- *Demonstrate on yourself.* Show your partner exactly what you like to do with your favorite sex toy. See "Masturbating with a Partner" in Chapter 5, "Masturbation."

- *Be playful.* We call them toys because they're meant to be fun! "My lover and I keep our lubes chilly in the fridge and then shock each other by dripping the cold lubricant on each other's steamy vaginas," wrote one woman.

- *Go shopping together.* Perhaps your partner isn't turned on by the toys you've got at home. You may be surprised by what catches her eye!

- *Talk about your misgivings.* Are you afraid you'll feel silly wearing a harness and dildo? Approach sex toys in the spirit of learning. "I have still have some work to do on my comfort level with strapping it on," wrote another. "But, you know, practice makes perfect!"

What are the most popular toys and accoutrements among lesbian and bisexual women customers of sex-toy boutiques? Happily, women's preferences are so varied and so individual that sex-toy popularity contests are worthless. So *what* if seven out of ten lesbians prefer that 8-inch silicone wonder—all that matters is whether it feels good to *you*. Still, a casual survey of toy saleswomen yields some interesting information.

The biggest recent innovations in sex toys are in materials, such as Cyberskin dildos, silicone lubes, glycerin-free lubes, and in the design of high-functioning "multitasking" toys, such as harnesses with a cuff to hold a dildo or butt plug inside the wearer, double dildos that really work, and vibrating anal probes with flexible spines.

Cyberskin is a new material that many women say feels just like skin. Made from a mixture of silicone and PVC (polyvinylchloride), Cyberskin dildos feature a hard core with a softer outer-layer. "Not only does Cyberskin quickly warm to body temperature, it's also very resilient—it can be stretched and pulled and will 'remember' its original shape," say the folks at Good Vibrations in San Francisco.[2]

"When Cyber Cock landed on our shelves," say the women of Come As You Are in Toronto, "it quickly became the must-have dildo. Its hyper-realistic look and feel made it the centerpiece of at least one dyke party we heard about. And the stampede began."[3]

The downside of Cyberskin is that it gets dirty—fast! The tacky surface attracts lint and other particles of dirt floating about your play space. That means that you really must use condoms with Cyberskin toys and clean them thoroughly after use. Since Cyberskin contains silicone, avoid use with silicone lube. See below, "How to Care for Your Toys."

Silicone lubricants like Eros Bodyglide, ID Millenium, and Wet Platinum are remarkably silky. They're slipperier than water-based lubes. They don't dry up or get sticky. They're never stringy. No wonder they've become so popular. They're condom-compatible, too; they contain no oils and won't destroy latex. Since they *do* last and last, you'll have to use soap and water to wash them off. Don't use silicone lube with silicone toys—the silicone in the lube may bond with the silicone in your toy, disfiguring your dildo. Silicone lubes are much more expensive than water-based lubes—but a little of it goes a long way.

Glycerin-free lube has proved to be a god(dess)-send to many women who experience yeast infections that can be traced to the glycerin contained in most water-based lubricants. Glycerin is similar in chemical composition to glucose—sugar—which can create a fertile environment for yeast infections to flourish.

Liquid Silk by Bodywise leads the pack of the new glycerin-free lubes. "Our customers rave about this creamy British lube," writes the Good Vibrations toy buyer. "It contains no glycerin and never gets sticky." [4] Liquid Silk is by far the best-selling lube at A Woman's Touch in Madison, Wisconsin. "For fisting and anal play, women tend to prefer Liquid Silk or its cousin, Maximus. It doesn't get sticky, has no smell, and feels close to the real thing." [5]

Double dildos have long been popular among women who are captivated by the fantasy of simultaneous vaginal penetration—but they rarely lived up to their promise. Either too floppy or too rigid, these double-headed dongs suffered from poor design. "Unfortunately the dream of the double-headed dildo often turns out to be impossible to realize," say the women of Toys in Babeland in Seattle and New York. Traditional models work for the few women who can "manage the scissors-like positioning and pulled shoulder muscles that come with the territory of a ruler-straight double." [6] Thankfully, new designs in double dildos have changed that scenario.

The Nexus is a harness-compatible silicone double dildo. It's 7 inches long and $1\frac{1}{2}$ inches in diameter at one end, and $6\frac{3}{4}$ inches long and $1\frac{1}{2}$ inches in diameter at the other end. According to A Woman's Touch, "Double dildos appeal to our customers because they allow the feeling of being connected. The Nexus is popular because it really is designed to work well (with the addition of a harness), and it provides clitoral stimulation to the wearer." [7]

Other recent innovations in multitasking include a pantheon of toys that provide additional stimulation during strap-on sex. Harness cuffs fasten onto the center strap of a thong-style harness to hold a dildo or butt plug inside the wearer of a strap-on dildo. Either partner can tuck any of a dozen small vibrators into a harness or pouch for clitoral stimulation during dildo play. (See "Fairy Butch's Stimulation Tips for Strap-On Sex" in Chapter 10, "Vaginal Penetration.")

Many toys try to do too much, with too little attention to design and engineering—they appeal to impulse rather than your "smart-shopper" savvy. The women of Toys in Babeland describe such toys as "huge, slimy, battery-powered monsters [that] will 'vibro twist' and 'corkscrew delight' their way right into your trashcan." [8]

I strap on a thick 7-inch vibrating jelly dildo. What a godsend! It seems to fit my partner's needs perfectly and the vibrating soft jelly-like texture feels absolutely fabulous on my clitoris.

There are exceptions, however—including vibrating jelly dildos and anal probes featuring flexible spines. One such toy is the Flex-O-Pleaser. "Yes, the name is dorkiness incarnate," say the folks at Blowfish, "but if you're looking for a vibrator for insertion play, we recommend this one highly." [9] This battery-operated vibrator features a 3-inch cylindrical head on a strong, flexible 5-inch shaft. The whole thing is attached to a 5-inch handle with an adjustable switch.

How to Choose Sex Toys

There are so many toys you can purchase or adapt for your pleasure, you may feel overwhelmed by the possibilities! A quick surfride through the web sites of retail and mail-order outlets will show a virtually limitless choice of sex toys. You can invent your own toys, making clever use of household items, or search the produce aisle of the grocery store for erotic inspiration. How can you find out what you like? A little window shopping will help, whether you browse on the Web or in person at your local sex-toy boutique. Here are some questions to consider as you begin your search, along with suggestions for play and cautions regarding safety. You can purchase the toys and supplies mentioned here from the mail-order and retail outlets listed in the "Resources" section.

Do You Like Clitoral Stimulation?

My Hitachi Magic Wand sends me into spiraling heights of orgasmic ecstasy! I like the Magic Wand because it's very fast and it can allow me to reach orgasm in a few minutes. It's like a quickie, but with a toy.

Vibrators provide steady, reliable clitoral stimulation. You can choose from electric vibrators, rechargeable vibrators, battery-operated vibrators, waterproof vibrators you can use in the bathtub, egg-shaped vibrators you can slip inside a harness cuff, and vibrators shaped like rabbits, beavers, and even bears!

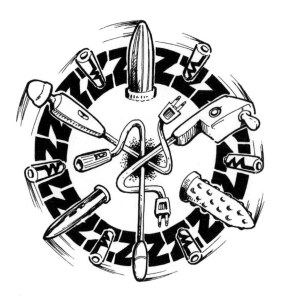

ILLUSTRATION 4. VIBRATORS

For an intense buzz, try a coil-operated electric vibrator, like the Wahl, which produces quite strong sensations and features a small point of contact that can focus sensation on a very small area. The all-time-best-selling Hitachi Magic Wand, with its tennis-ball-shaped head, produces somewhat more diffuse sensations, though you can slip an attachment over the head for more specifically focused vibrations.

Battery-operated vibrators tend to produce sensations that are less intense than those of electric vibrators. They also don't hold up to years of use, unlike many electric vibrators. However, they come in many more shapes and styles than electric vibrators and are much less expensive. Battery-operated vibrators are quite versatile—they're easily adapted to use with dildos and harnesses as well as other toys. Plus they'll fit in your pocket, purse, backpack, suitcase, and the glove compartment of your car. See Chapter 8, "Clitoral Play."

> *For solo delights, I like the Rabbit Pearl, a rotating dildo with revolving "pearls"*
> *in the shaft and two vibrating bunny ears that fit on either side of my clit.... Yum!*

Do You Like Nipple Stimulation?

You may enjoy playing with clothespins, tweezer and alligator clamps, tit pumps, suction cups, hot wax, piercing needles, and other toys. Try wetting your nipple with lube and then caressing it as you would your clitoris. See Chapter 7, "Breast Play," and "Teach Yourself Some New Tricks" in Chapter 13, "Play Nice! (or Else…)."

Sex and Disability: Toy Accessibility

The folks at Come As You Are in Toronto are dedicated to making sex accessible to everyone—including people with disabilities. Their web site is packed with specific information on making sex toys accessible for disabled customers. Here's their advice:

Make your sex toys your own—be inventive in adapting and playing with your toys. Of course, no toy will be perfect for everyone. If you want help adapting your toys, consult an occupational therapist. Although some occupational therapists may not share your sexual politics (and may even blush at your request to build up the handle on your vibrator), they do have the training and materials to help you make your sex toys more functional.

Consider the weight, size, and shape of the toy. If you can't hold a toy in your hand, try a vibrator that fits in a pouch, such as the Leather Butterfly. The straps fit around your waist and between your legs. You may also be able to use a larger electric vibrator by positioning yourself beside it. Be careful not to lie directly on top of a vibrator, as this will cut off the ventilation for the motor and can be very dangerous.

If you're able to hold a toy, but tire easily, choose something lightweight. Consider the fact that, all things considered, you may be distracted while holding the toy. Some vibrators fit on the hand, which provides a little more support. You can wear an egg-shaped vibe in a glove. The only thing more annoying than your batteries dying at exactly the wrong time is dropping the toy!

Consider the material of the toy. If you have allergies, environmental sensitivities, or a reduced immune system, stay away from products with heavy scents. Many people have allergies to latex. A lot of toys are made primarily of nonlatex rubber products. However, even "nonlatex" products may contain some latex. If you have a very sensitive latex allergy, stick with hard plastic or silicone toys.

Consider the switch on an electric or battery-operated toy. This is often the most aggravating part of buying toys. Manufacturers tend not to think about accessibility, and it shows in their switches. Some toys are easy to turn on and off and others are not. If you find a toy you love with a difficult switch, you may be able to find someone to rig an accessible switch.

Choose a toy with a long reach, such as the Flex-O-Pleaser..

Vibrating cock rings fit snugly on the fingers. The jelly rubber rings are especially nice; the rubber extension provides a little extra support as you press the vibrator against your body.

Thigh Harness and Night Rider: The Thigh Harness is particularly good for people with lower back problems who find their back gives out before they do. The Night Rider, which straps onto furniture, is an incredibly versatile harness and comes with some ten feet of extra cord.

Do You Like Vaginal Penetration?

My favorite toy is my slender, curving, purple-and-black-swirled silicone dildo, Champ. I think its form is elegant, and its coloring beautiful. It's just the right size for me when I'm really hot and loose.

Dildos come in all sizes and shapes—from the diminutive 5-inch Pal to the meaty 10-inch Prince. You'll find dildos in silicone, rubber, Cyberskin, and other materials. Dildos are available in a variety of colors—black, lavender, and swirl patterns, among many others. You no longer need to put up with a sickly pinkish hue marketed as "flesh tone" (which one savvy retailer calls DOA Caucasian!). You can buy dildos in a variety of abstract designs, realistic dildos with veins and balls, dildos shaped like dolphins, double dildos, battery-operated vibrating dildos, and dildos with slits in their base to fit a small egg-shaped vibrator.

Do you like deep thrusting rather than a feeling of fullness? Try a long, slender dildo. Make sure it's firm enough to stay rigid. Do you like a feeling of being stretched wide? You might like a thick, squat dildo.

I love my amethyst Jelly Jewel. It's a bit too long (10 inches) but it's the perfect width—almost two inches. It's realistic—it doesn't apologize for its invasive attitude.

Dildos are sold by diameter and length. For strap-on sex, you'll want a dildo at least an inch or two longer than one you'd use by hand, since the harness and your body will absorb some length. You can "measure" your vagina with a zucchini or cucumber. Experiment with vegetables of varying length and girth; when you find a vegetable of a thickness that suits you, cut it lengthwise in half. You can now measure the diameter. Dildo length is measured from the base to the tip. Even if you shop organically, remember to slip a condom over that cucumber!

You can also experiment with dildos by purchasing inexpensive rubber models. When you find the length, girth, shape, and style you like, you can then invest in a high-quality silicone dildo. Remember that you *must* use condoms on rubber dildos, since they're more porous than silicone and will absorb dirt very easily. See Chapter 10, "Vaginal Penetration."

Do You Like G-Spot Stimulation?

Any curved, firm insertive toy is a candidate for
G-spot stimulation. Of course, whether or not it
hits the spot will vary from woman to woman.
Some women get the best results from G-spot
attachments designed to fit over the head of an
electric vibrator, such as the G-Spotter for the
Hitachi Magic Wand. Others prefer insertable
vibrators with rotating shafts, or dildos with ridges
or a prominent, cock-like head. The all-time
classic G-spot toy is the Crystal Wand, which
Toys in Babeland describes as "10 inches of clear
acrylic hand molded into a shallow S-shape."[10]
See Chapter 3, "Anatomy and Sexual Response,"
for more on your G-spot.

Do You Like Anal Penetration?

> I have a fairly small silicone butt plug. I like
> how it warms to my body and is flexible so that
> it doesn't tear or otherwise brutalize me. It's
> great for added zing during almost any sexual
> activity.

Butt plugs are popular toys for anal penetration. Butt plugs aren't intended for thrusting.
They're designed to be held inside your rectum
by your sphincter muscles. Like dildos, butt plugs
come in all shapes and sizes—from the minia-
ture Flirt (which is hardly bigger than your
index finger) to the great big Triple Ripple plugs
(which dwarf your fist)—and in a variety of
materials. Again, if you're not sure what size or

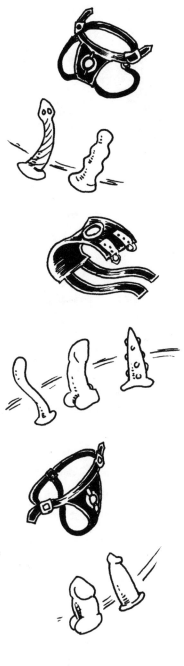

**ILLUSTRATION 5.
DILDOS AND HARNESSES**

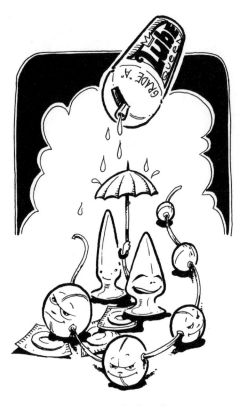

ILLUSTRATION 6. ANAL TOYS

style you'll like, buy a cheap rubber plug before graduating to higher-quality silicone. Don't forget that what may seem rather diminutive when placed on the counter at your local toy store may seem humongous when placed inside your rectum at home.

Jelly dildos are a great choice for anal penetration, since the soft rubber won't abrade delicate rectal tissues. At Grand Opening in Brookline, Massachusetts, the most popular vibrating anal toy is the Butt Buzzer, which combines "wonderful flexible jelly rubber" with a silver "pearl" vibrator embedded in its shaft.[11] Of course, women are very individual in their choice of materials for anal toys—you might prefer a heavy chrome butt plug to a jelly dildo!

Don't overlook anal beads, vibrating butt plugs, flexible anal probes, and other toys specifically designed for butt play. See Chapter 11, "Anal Penetration."

The rules for anal toys bear repeating here:

- The toy must have a flared base to prevent it from slipping inside your rectum and working its way into the colon. Similarly, anal beads must be securely fastened to their string and have a ring on the end to hold onto.
- The toy must have a smooth surface—no sharp edges or breakable parts.
- You must be able to clean the toy with antibacterial soap and hot water.
- If you intend to use the toy to penetrate your partner deeply, it must be flexible enough to maneuver the curves of the rectum.
- Use lots of lube! Since the rectum isn't self-lubricating like the vagina, make sure you coat your toy thoroughly with lube.

Do You Want to Strap On Your Dildo?

I definitely like the ability to strap it on. It leaves both of my hands free to use on other parts of her body. There is no better feeling in the world, for me, than to wrap my arms around her while I am penetrating her as she reaches orgasms.

Dildo harnesses come in several styles and materials. They can strap onto your hips, your thigh, a chair—or even your face. Choose your harness to fit both the dildo you wish to use with it and the style of sex play you prefer.

- *What size dildo do you want to use?* Any dildo with a flared base can be worn with a harness—if it's not too thick to fit through the cock ring or opening in the harness! The key is selecting the right harness. The Terra Firma harness comes with three rubber cock rings that snap into place. Theoretically, you could swap these for any size cock ring and thus any dildo with a flared base—even the 2-inch-diameter Prince. The Crown harness also can be adapted to use with large or small dildos. Other harnesses have a fixed cock ring or a reinforced hole through which the dildo protrudes. For instance, Aslan harnesses have a standard $1\,^3/_4$ inch hole. Your choice of dildo is limited by the diameter of the hole. If you intend to wear your harness with a variety of dildos, you'd do well to select a harness with a detachable cock ring or an adjustable opening.
- *What kind of material do you like?* You can find well-constructed harnesses in leather, vinyl, rubber, and nylon webbing. Nylon is less expensive than leather, of course, and quite sturdy.
- *Do you want to strap on additional penetrative toys?* If you want to use a cuff to hold a butt plug or dildo inside the wearer, select a harness with a center strap.
- *What's your hip size?* The Crown harness works well for women of substantial size. Since the harness rides high on the wearer's hips, her belly won't get in the way of deep penetration. The Crown comes in hip sizes up to 60 inches. Aslan Leather makes harnesses that accommodate hip sizes up to 38 inches, but they'll customize their designs to fit larger women. Stormy Leather's Texas Two-Strap and Terra Firma harnesses fit hips up to 46 inches.

- *Are you curious about other ways to strap on a dildo?* In addition to harnesses you wear around your hip, you can also try a thigh harness, a harness you strap onto a chair, and even a face harness, which lets a dildo protrude from your mouth or forehead (in a 69 position, you can penetrate your partner vaginally while performing cunnilingus). You can even try a dildo harness that doubles as a chastity belt. Aslan Leather offers a model with the standard hole for the protruding dildo, two extra holes for vaginal and anal penetration of the wearer, a studded leather crotch piece—and the whole thing locks in three places!

Do You Want to Explore Gender Play?

My favorite is a Cyberskin dildo. He's almost 8 inches long and made of very realistic material, complete with balls that are actually two balls inside a scrotum. Unfortunately, he's not rigid enough to be used for serious fucking, but I love him just the same.

Sometimes a cigar is *not* just a cigar! If you want a dildo you can wear as a cock, check out these models:

- *Want a realistic feel?* Cyberskin now comes in several models—the basic realistic dildo, a vibrating version, and a stretchy sleeve you can pull over any dildo or cylindrical vibe.
- *Want a realistic look?* Realistic dildos feature detailed glans, veins, and balls. You can emulate Jeff Stryker with a dildo modeled after the porn star himself. Or try the Johnny—7 $1/2$ inches long and 2 inches in diameter. Why would a lesbian buy a dildo with balls? Aside from the realistic look and feel, the balls

Packing somehow completes me.
It makes me feel real.

provide extra stimulation for the receptive partner—when thrusting in a rear-entry position, they slap against her vulva.

- *Do you pack?* You might enjoy the Pack 'n Play, a semihard 5-inch dildo that creates a realistic bulge in your pants. While the name suggests that you might want to also use this dildo for penetration, you might not find it hard enough for serious play. Cyberskin dildos bend easily enough to tuck into your briefs. You'll find a variety of dildos made from soft "fleshy" material— comfortable enough to wear under clothing, plus you won't look like you've got a baseball bat in your pants!

Do You Want to Explore BDSM?

You'll find discussion of a number of BDSM toys and devices in Chapter 13, "Play Nice! (or Else…)." Make sure your toys are well made and come from reputable sources. Many makers of whips and other S/M toys are truly artisans; as Janette Heartwood says, their passion for the erotic exchange of power translates into their products. [12] Some of the mail-order and retail outlets listed in "Resources" have fabulous web sites with photos of toys (and gorgeous women models!). Others offer print catalogs. Blowfish, JT's Stockroom, and Purple Passion, among others, carry a full line of bondage and S/M toys. Some web sites offer helpful information on toy care and safety as well.

Do You Want to Explore New Fantasies?

Porn! Whether you rent an explicit video, read a collection of erotic fiction, or surf erotica web sites, you'll find that porn can fuel your imagination. What do lesbians look for in video porn? Tastes vary: Hard core. Soft core. Tranny porn. Girl–girl. Girl–boy. Boy–boy. Some lesbians prefer gay male porn for its raw depictions of sexuality.

Whether looking for images of tenderness and romance or down-and-dirty back alley sex, lesbians want authenticity. Having viewed a glut of mainstream porn featuring heterosexual-appearing actresses, lesbians want to see "authentic pleasure and chemistry between the performers," as one Good Vibrations saleswoman wrote. [13] You'll find a selection of lesbian porn titles in the "Resources" guide.

Got Your Lube?

I love Probe Thin and Silky because it dries quickly without being sticky. It also doesn't taste bad and feels soooo slick when rubbed on me.

Lube is the most essential item in your toy bag. Not only will lubricant make sex more pleasurable, it will keep you from getting raw during vaginal penetration. For anal penetration, lube is a *must*—the rectum is not self-lubricating, and the friction of a finger or dildo thrusting in and out could tear the delicate tissue.

Everyone has an opinion about lube. While one woman loves Probe, another will swear by ID Liquid, or Astroglide, or Wet. How do you find out which lube you might like? If your local pharmacy stocks only one brand of lube and the nearest sex-toy store is 200 miles away, order a sampler pack from one of the retail or mail-order outlets listed in the "Resources." You'll get a variety of little plastic "pillows" containing just enough lube for one use (sufficient for clitoral stimulation, but certainly not enough for fisting!). When you decide which brand of lube you prefer, you can order more economical sizes. These individual-sized packets are great for travel and for group sex—you won't end up with many sticky fingers handling the same bottle (shared lube containers, like shared sex toys, can lead to transmission of many STDs).

Most lube manufacturers offer a full line of water-based lubes, including a silky, light lube for clitoral play or vaginal penetration, and a thick, viscous lube for anal penetration and vaginal fisting. Here are some questions to think about when choosing lube:

- *Will you engage in clitoral play?* Try a thin, light lube such as ID Liquid, Probe Silky Light, Astroglide, Liquid Silk, or Eros Bodyglide.
- *Will you engage in vaginal penetration?* Some women prefer a light lube, others a more viscous lube, like Slippery Stuff, Maximus, and Probe for penetration.
- *Will you engage in vaginal fisting?* Buy the pump bottle! You may want to try a thicker lube, like Probe Thick and Rich.
- *Will you engage in anal penetration?* Try ForPlay, Maximus, Probe Classic, or Slippery Stuff for a thicker water-based lube. Some women use oil-based lube,

such as Crisco or Elbow Grease, for anal play; be careful, though, that the lube doesn't drip into the vagina. Oil deteriorates latex; you'll have to change your latex glove every 15 minutes. If you use an oil-based lube with a latex condom-covered toy, plan on disinfecting the toy. The oil in the lube will have destroyed the latex.

- *Will you engage in oral sex?* If you anticipate oral contact as well as penetration, choose a lube that's tasteless, such as ID or Probe, or intended for oral play—such as the flavored lubes from Wet or ForPlay. Avoid lubes containing nonoxynol-9, which will numb your tongue and lips.
- *Will you be using latex?* Any water-based or silicone lube will be compatible with your latex gloves and condoms. Avoid oil-based lubes (see above).
- *Will you be using silicone toys?* Don't use silicone lube with silicone dildos. The silicone in the lube will degrade your silicone toy.
- *Do you get yeast infections?* Choose a glyercin-free lube such as Liquid Silk, or its thicker counterpart, Maximus.
- *Do you want a lube that will last and last?* Silicone lubes such as Eros Bodyglide and Wet Platinum won't dry up or get sticky.
- *Are you sensitive to chemicals?* Avoid lubes containing nonoxynol-9, a detergent added to lubricants as a spermicide.

Got Your Safer-Sex Supplies?
Stock your toy bag with these basic safer-sex supplies:
- Latex, vinyl, or nitrile gloves for penetrative sex.
- Finger cots, which are like little finger-sized condoms. You may have noticed that I've said nothing about finger cots in this book. Since a caress of a fingertip often leads to more—a second finger, the palm of the hand—I find that finger cots have limited use and recommend gloves instead.
- Condoms to cover dildos, butt plugs, and vibrators.
- Dental dams, Lollyes, or plastic wrap for cunnilingus and rimming.
- Hibiclens, antibacterial hand soap, or a toy cleaner such as ForPlay Adult Toy Cleanser to clean dildos, vibrator attachments, lube bottles, and other toys after use. Wash your hands with antibacterial soap.

- Alcohol wipes to clean handles of vibrators and other toys, as well as for use in play piercing and other activities where blood may be present.
- A simple first aid kit, including antiseptic ointment, bandages, adhesive tape, and scissors.

Does Latex Make You Itch?

If you notice a rash after wearing a latex glove, you may be developing a sensitivity to latex. Some women are so allergic to latex that they develop hives, become nauseated, or have trouble breathing when they come into contact with latex products.

Who's at risk for latex allergies? People who come into frequent or continual contact with latex. Health care workers are especially at risk. Not only do they snap gloves on and off all day long, their work environment is permeated by the fumes given off by latex products. Add safer-sex practices to that scenario and you can see why licking a latex Lollye could be a nightmare for a latex-sensitive woman.

The only solution to latex sensitivity is to avoid latex as much as possible. Here are some alternatives:

- Nitrile gloves contain no latex, and they're thinner than most latex gloves. They can be used with water-based, oil-based, and silicone lubricants. They're more expensive than latex, however. Vinyl gloves are also an alternative to latex.
- Plastic wrap is a cheap alternative to latex dams.
- Polyurethane condoms by Avanti are an alternative to latex condoms. They're thinner and larger than latex condoms and can be used with water-based, oil-based, and silicone lubricants. However, they are much more expensive than latex condoms. *Do not* use lambskin condoms for safer sex; they won't prevent transmission of viruses such as HIV.

Latex-free safer sex supplies are available from Cetra Latex-Free Supplies, as well as other mail order and retail outlets listed in the "Resources."

How's Your Budget?

If you want to have fun on a budget, try some of these suggestions:

- Buy latex gloves by the box. Most large pharmacies have a house brand.
- Get your condoms for free at gay bars and events sponsored by AIDS prevention organizations. Safeguarding your health is as important as safeguarding anyone else's.
- Use plastic wrap, cut-up gloves, or condoms for dental dams.
- Keep a spray bottle of water by your bed. Rather than continuously adding more water-based lube, spray a little water on your glove or dildo to reactivate the lube.
- If you like silicone or gylcerin-free lubes, look for the cheaper brands. Eros Bodyglide and Liquid Silk are so popular as to have spawned less-expensive imitations.
- Buy cheap rubber dildos and butt plugs—they cost half as much as their silicone counterparts. You can hide their less-than-pleasing look and texture under a condom.
- Nylon harnesses cost less than leather and will do the job quite well.
- Some BDSM toy vendors cater to customers who want to stock their play rooms inexpensively. Certain toys, such as canes and crops, lend themselves to economizing, while others don't—cheap whips are just that: cheap. Use your imagination—a wooden spoon makes a great paddle; a chair works well as a bondage station.

How to Care for Your Toys

Clean your toys with warm water and soap—preferably antibacterial soap, Hibiclens, or a toy cleaner such as ForPlay Adult Toy Cleanser. Never submerge electric or battery-operated toys in water.

Silicone can be cleaned by boiling for two to three minutes. You can also clean silicone dildos in your dishwasher. Keep silicone lubricants away from silicone toys.

Rubber dildos are more porous than silicone and will absorb dirt. Always use condoms with rubber dildos, and clean them thoroughly with soap and water after each use.

Cyberskin is a challenge to keep clean—always use condoms with Cyberskin dildos. The skin-like surface attracts dirt. Cyberskin toys can't be cleaned by boiling, so use soap and water, dry thoroughly, and dust with corn starch. (*Do not* use baby powder or talc, which has been linked to cervical cancer.)

Nylon harnesses can be washed in the sink—or you can toss them into the washing machine. Hang to dry.

Clean leather harnesses with soap and water and hang dry. To disinfect, wipe with a cloth soaked in 70 percent isopropyl alcohol and then wipe clean with soap and water. After cleaning, use a leather conditioner to prevent the leather from drying out (never hang in the sun).

To clean a leather flogger, wipe each tail individually with a damp cloth soaked in either soap and water or leather cleaner, such as Lexol. To disinfect, wipe with a cloth soaked in 70 percent isopropyl alcohol and then wipe clean with soap and water. Don't store leather until it's completely dry to avoid mold. Use a leather conditioner to prevent the leather from drying out.

Suggested Web Links:

COME AS YOU ARE
www.comeasyouare.com
GOOD VIBRATIONS
www.goodvibes.com
PURPLE PASSION
www.purplepassion.com

NOTES

1. Good Vibrations web site, www.goodvibes.com
2. Good Vibrations, product insert.
3. Sarah Forbes-Roberts and Sandra Haar, Come As You Are, correspondence.
4. Sarah Dewhirst, Good Vibrations, correspondence.
5. Ellen Barnard, A Woman's Touch, correspondence.
6. Rachel Venning, Toys in Babeland, "I Dream of Dildos," *Girlfriends Magazine*, vol. 1, no. 1, July 1994, 32.
7. Ellen Barnard, A Woman's Touch, correspondence.
8. Rachel Venning, Toys in Babeland, "I Dream of Dildos"
9. Blowfish Web site, www.blowfish.com
10. Toys in Babeland, "The Crystal Wand," *Girlfriends Magazine*, vol. 4, no. 6, October 1997, 40.
11. Grand Opening web site, www.grandopening.com
12. Janette Heartwood, Heartwood Whips of Passion, web page, www.heartwoodwhips.com
13. Terry Morris, Good Vibrations, correspondence.

SOURCE OF SIDEBAR

"Toy Accessibility" is adapted from the Come As You are web site, www.comeasyouare.com

chapter sixteen

Safer Sex and Gynecological Health

I have herpes. I'm very up front about it.

DO YOU THINK THAT IF YOU'RE NOT SEXUALLY ACTIVE WITH MEN, you're not at risk for STDs? If so, you're not alone! Many lesbians think that living an exclusively "lesbian lifestyle" immunizes them against sexually transmitted conditions—and, for that matter, most gynecological concerns. Not so!

Unfortunately, when it comes to sexually transmitted diseases, some health care practitioners think the same thing. Knowing very little about lesbian sexual practices, they make assumptions—that lesbians don't have penetrative sex, or anal sex, or that lesbians don't have sex at all.

More troubling, those who research STD transmission may not know much about lesbian sex either. They may use terms like "oral sex" and "vaginal intercourse" in safer-sex guidelines without defining them. Does oral sex refer to cunnilingus? Or just fellatio? Does penetration with a dildo count as "intercourse"? How do you know what's safe?

Few clinical studies have been conducted of woman-to-woman transmission of STDs. Can chlamydia be transmitted by sharing a dildo with an infected partner? Can you give your partner herpes or trichomoniasis through frottage? Can you get HIV by going down on a menstruating woman who has the virus? What about hepatitis? A cautious physician will tell you that, yes, all of these scenarios are quite possible—but that not enough studies have been done to offer conclusive answers.

Since women who have sex with women are often left out of health research, our health care needs are neglected. Jeanne Marrazzo, of the Lesbian-Bisexual Women's Health Study at the University of Washington, says that because "lesbians do not fit the very narrowly and poorly defined risk profile, they are being told that as lesbian/bisexual women they do not need Pap smears or STD screenings."[1]

None of which inspires confidence when you're sitting on the examination table in a paper gown and your health care practitioner cheerfully asks whether you're sexually "active" and what kind of birth control you use. No wonder few of us feel comfortable speaking candidly about our sexual histories and practices.

But if medical research skirts the issue of woman-to-woman transmission of STDs, and if you don't feel comfortable coming out to a physician, how will your gynecologist know what to look for?

Talking to Your Doctor About Sex

As Tristan Taormino says, "Your gynecological visit is no time to play 'Don't Ask, Don't Tell.' If they don't ask, it's your responsibility to tell."[2] It's important for your health that you come out to your health caregiver. Find a physician you feel comfortable with. Look for someone you think you can talk to. Even a lesbian gynecologist can't guess what you do in bed.

You can't rely on your health care practitioner to make you feel comfortable talking about sex. Physicians trained in the United States receive only 12 hours instruction in human sexuality. Your doctor may be even less comfortable than you discussing the details of your sex life—especially if your physician sees few other lesbian, bisexual, or transgendered patients.

Charles Moser, author of *Health Care Without Shame: A Handbook for the Sexually Diverse and Their Caregivers*, recommends that you come out to your physician during your first visit—if not sooner.[3] Don't wait until you suspect you have an STD. What should you tell your health care practitioner about your sex life? Here are some of the points Moser suggests you cover:

- The sexual activities you typically engage in—such as oral sex, vaginal or anal penetration with fingers or a dildo, or fisting.
- The safer sex precautions you employ.
- The number of partners with whom you have sexual contact.
- Whether you engage in activities that might involve bruising or breaking the skin (such as caning or play piercing).
- The family structures or relationships you wish have taken into account for hospital visitation or decisions regarding your care. [4]

Finally, if you don't feel comfortable follwing Moser's recommendations, some health advocates suggest you simply say that you are sexually active and want to be tested for the full spectrum of STDs.

Gynecological Care

All sexually active females should get annual gynecological exams, including Pap smear, pelvic exam, and breast exam. Whether you have sex with one partner or many, with women only or with both women and men, you need regular gynecological care. Regardless of your gender identity—stone butches require gynecological care, too!

If you engage in unprotected sexual activities, ask to be screened for STDs. If you engage in anal sex, ask for a rectal exam—some STDs can infect you rectally as well as genitally. As you'll see below, STDs often occur without any symptoms—or with symptoms you could easily mistake for the flu! A Pap smear, blood test, or culture may be the only way you know you've been exposed to an STD.

If you're diagnosed with an STD or have had an abnormal Pap smear, your physician will recommend treatment. It's important that you follow up on recommended procedures and return visits. Your annual Pap smear can prevent cervical cancer *only* if you treat any dysplasia or other conditions revealed by the test!

Consult a gynecologist if you experience pain during penetrative sex or if you experience spotting after deep thrusting with a dildo, fingers, or fist. You may have a small tear or abrasion on your cervix.

If you notice a rash or sore on your genitals or anus, unusual discharge, or irregular bleeding, or if you experience genital itchiness or irritation, painful urination, abdominal or pelvic pain, nausea, fatigue, or fever, consult a physician. Don't ignore these symptoms.

STDs and Gynecological Concerns

Many gynecological problems can be easily cleared up. Left untreated, they can lead to very serious health problems. Bacterial STDs can be treated with antibiotics. Viral STDs can't be "cured"—but there are medications to alleviate outbreaks, as with herpes, as well as new treatment protocols for HIV that have been effective for many people.

"Latex provides protection on whatever surface it is covering," say the researchers on LesbianSTD.com.[5] Use of latex on insertive sex toys such as dildos and vibrators prevents transmission of bacterial STDs like chlamydia and gonorrhea. Use of plastic wrap or latex gloves on skin prevents transmission of viruses like herpes and HPV. Saran wrap is considered a better barrier for oral sex than conventional dental dams, which are too small. Of course, if you do have sex with men (penis-vagina, penis-anus or fellatio), use a condom. (See Chapter 4, "The Road to Heaven Leads to You," for a complete list of safer-sex guidelines.)

Here are some STDs and other gynecological conditions you should know about:

Allergies and chemical sensitivity. While allergies aren't sexually transmitted conditions, they certainly will affect your sex life! The vaginal discharge, itching, and irritation they cause may lead you to mistake allergic vaginosis for a yeast infection. You may be sensitive to latex, the powder used on latex gloves, glycerin in a particular brand of lubricant, spermicides, or microbicides like nonoxynol-9, or other products. The best treatment is to discontinue use of the irritant. See Chapter 15, "Sex Toys and Accoutrements," for information on lubricants, latex allergies, and alternative safer-sex supplies.

Nonoxynol-9 is a detergent that's added to some lubricants (including some lubricated condoms) to kill the HIV virus. Many women find nonoxynol-9

LesbianSTD.com

When I first logged onto LesbianSTD.com, I wanted to leap out of my chair. Finally, a Web site addressing *my* safer-sex concerns. Here are some things I learned:

- Human papillomavirus (HPV), one of the most common STDs, can cause genital warts and abnormal Pap smears, and in some women can lead to cervical cancer.

- HPV can be transmitted from one woman to another.

- Bacterial vaginosis (BV) is strongly associated with preterm labor and low birth weight.

- BV is often diagnosed in both partners in lesbian couples.

- Both HPV and BV have been seen in many lesbians and bisexual women, even those with no prior sexual history with men.

- Medical literature contains case reports of woman-to-woman transmission of HIV. The most likely sources of transmission are menstrual blood, vaginal discharge when there is vaginitis (more white blood cells containing HIV may be present then), and traumatic sex practices.

---

irritating to the mucous membranes of the vagina and rectum. There is much debate regarding the use of nonoxynol-9. Some sex educators and physicians recommend nonoxynol-9 for use with condoms during penis-to-vagina and penis-to-anus penetration as added insurance against HIV transmission.[6] Others argue that the irritations caused by nonoxynol-9 outweigh the benefits. Especially regarding anal sex, they recommend that you *not* use nonoxynol-9.[7] Irritating the delicate rectal tissue, they argue, can encourage HIV transmission by providing the virus with an accessible route to the bloodstream. In fact, a study of nonoxynol-9 use among women sex workers in South Africa showed that genital lesions caused by the chemical may result in increased HIV transmission risk.[8]

However, Jeanne Marrazzo differs with these conclusions. She feels that nonoxynol-9 can help prevent woman-to woman transmission of STDs with little risk of vaginal ulceration—providing that it's used in moderation. She cautions that women discontinue use of nonoxynol-9 if any irritation develops.[9]

Bacterial vaginosis. This condition may be transmitted sexually between women with such frequency that one researcher calls BV an "STD among lesbians." [10] One study of lesbian health reported an 80 percent concurrence rate for bacterial vaginosis among monogamous lesbian couples. [11] Yet, it has not been medically proven that bacterial vaginosis, caused by an imbalance of bacteria normally found in the vagina, is, in fact, sexually transmitted at all. [12] Still, partners should be evaluated. If you notice a yellowish vaginal discharge, vaginal itching or irritation, or a strong odor, you may have a vaginal infection. Bacterial vaginosis is treated with antibiotics. Use only water-based lubricants in the vagina; oil-based lubes are difficult to wash out. Do not allow anal bacteria entry into the vagina. Change gloves when you move from anal to vaginal penetration—or wash your hands with an antibacterial soap. Use condoms on shared sex toys. Change condoms when you change activities or partners.

Chlamydia and gonorrhea. According to the Lesbian-Bisexual Women's Health Study, woman-to-woman transmission of chlamydia and gonorrhea "seems to be rare," though such transmission is possible. [13] Why don't we know how frequently women transmit chlamydia and gonorrhea to each other? Jeanne Marrazzo thinks this is a problem of surveillance and reporting. Both chlamydia and gonorrhea infect the cervix and can be transmitted through penetrative sex. Researchers, she says, assume that lesbians don't have penetrative sex. (Interestingly, 147 of the 149 women in Marrazzo's study of HPV in woman who have sex with women, had penetrative vaginal sex with women in the year prior to the study! [14]) In fact, Marrazzo believes that chlamydia and gonorrhea can be transmitted by dildos and hands. According to her, a shared dildo can carry chlamydia and gonorrhea from cervix to cervix, as can an unwashed hand. If you engage in fisting and then touch yourself, you could acquire chlamydia or gonorrhea. [15] Wash your hands with bacterial soap when changing partners or sexual activities—and before you touch yourself. [16] Use condoms or gloves on shared sex toys and gloves on your hands.

With 4 million new infections each year, some health educators are calling chlamydia the "silent epidemic" because it's so frequently asymptomatic. [17] In fact, most women with chlamydia have no symptoms. Others may notice a yellowish vaginal discharge, painful urination, abdominal pain, or irregular bleeding. Untreated, chlamydia can lead to pelvic inflammatory disease (PID), a cause of infertility. Chlamydia is caused by the *chlamydia trachomatis* bacteria and is treated with antibiotics.

Symptoms of gonorrhea are similar to chlamydia—vaginal discharge, irregular bleeding, and PID symptoms. As with chlamydia, it's possible to have gonorrhea without symptoms. Gonorrhea is caused by *neisseria gonorrheae* bacteria and is treated with antibiotics.

Hepatitis is an inflammation of the liver most commonly caused by three virus strains: hepatitis A virus (HAV), hepatitis B virus (HBV), and hepatitis C virus (HCV). Symptoms include fatigue, depression, nausea, loss of appetite, fever, chills, stomach pain, body aches, diarrhea, weight loss, headaches, and jaundice. Some people carry the hepatitis virus without having any symptoms at all. Hepatitis is diagnosed through a blood test. For many people, hepatitis is a lifelong chronic illness. If you have hepatitis B or C, don't share toothbrushes, razors, or piercing/cutting instruments, and don't expose partners to your menstrual blood .

Hepatitis A (HAV). You can transmit or acquire hepatitis A through unprotected rimming—regardless of the gender of your partners. If you engage in unprotected rimming, consider getting a vaccination for hepatitis A and use a latex barrier or plastic wrap for rimming.

Hepatitis B (HBV). You can transmit or acquire hepatitis B through cunnilingus, especially during menstruation. Hepatitis B is more likely to be transmitted through sharing needles for IV drug use, tattooing or piercing, and accidental needle sticks. If you engage in unprotected cunnilingus with

Talking about sex histories and negotiating safer sex has improved my sex life, because I feel closer to my partner— and we also talk about what turns us on.

menstruating partners, or if you engage in *any* activities where blood contact is possible, consider getting a vaccination for hepatitis B. Use a latex barrier or plastic wrap for cunnilingus.

Hepatitis C (HCV). It's estimated that more than 5 million people in the United States are infected with hepatitis C—and perhaps as many as 200 million worldwide. In most cases, hepatitis C is asymptomatic for years, even decades, before progressing to chronic liver disease. Many people who are infected with hepatitis C don't know they have it. Clearly, hepatitis C is epidemic. [18]

The risk of sexual transmission of hepatitis C hasn't been determined, though the risk is probably higher if you engage in S/M blood play or come into contact with blood during sex. Hepatitis C *may be* transmitted through woman-to-woman sex involving cunnilingus during menstruation. Hepatitis C is most often transmitted through sharing needles for IV drug use, tattooing or piercing, and accidental needle sticks. Use dental dams or other barriers to prevent transmission during cunnilingus. There's no vaccination for hepatitis C.

Herpes. An estimated 150 million people in the United States have been exposed to the herpes-2 virus. [19] Herpes is a chronic, viral STD that's extremely contagious:

- Most people with herpes don't know they have it.
- Many believe that the virus can be spread only during an outbreak—which is not true. The herpes virus may be shedding even when there are no visible symptoms.
- Herpes can be transmitted through skin-to-skin contact, including frottage (without clothing), hand-to-vulva and hand-to-anus contact.
- Herpes sores can break out not only *on* the genitals but in the area *surrounding* the genitals. Condoms and dental dams may not cover a large enough area to prevent transmission during outbreaks.
- Herpes can be transmitted from one mucosal membrane to another—from mouth to vulva and from vulva to mouth. As the receptive partner in cunnilingus, you can get genital herpes from a partner who has oral herpes. As the partner performing cunnilingus, you can get oral herpes from a partner who has genital herpes.

Herpes is caused by one of two viruses: *herpes simplex type 1* (HSV-1), which is oral herpes; or *herpes simplex type 2* (HSV-2), which is genital herpes. Prior to a herpes outbreak, you may experience flu-like symptoms or itching and tingling in the affected area. You may develop a very painful, raw herpes blister in the affected area. Outbreaks can be brought on by stress or a compromised immune system. Health care providers diagnose genital herpes by visual inspection and by testing a tissue sample from the sore. While there's no cure for herpes, there are medications that can help prevent or alleviate outbreaks. Use gloves on hands for finger fucking and fisting, and plastic wrap for oral sex. Cover sex toys with a condom or glove. Change condoms and gloves between partners.

HIV (human immunodeficiency virus) is transmitted when semen, blood, vaginal fluids, or breast milk of an infected person enter the bloodstream. Small lacerations or abrasions in the mouth, anus, vagina, or skin can provide a route for transmission of the HIV virus. Sores from herpes or other STDs can also provide a way for the HIV virus to enter the bloodstream, which is why having certain STDs can increase your risk for HIV.

Since HIV is present in both blood and vaginal secretions, it's possible to transmit HIV through unprotected cunnilingus, particularly when the receptive partner is menstruating and the other has bleeding gums or sores in her mouth. Although few in number, cases have been reported of woman-to-woman sexual transmission of HIV. More commonly, women who have sex with women acquire HIV through IV drug use, sperm donor insemination, or sex with men.

Understanding the potential for woman-to-woman transmission is complicated by the fact that models for reporting incidents of HIV infection don't account for lesbian sex. An HIV-positive lesbian or bisexual woman with other risk behaviors (for example, unprotected anal intercourse with men, injection drug use, needle use for piercing and tattooing, or use of unscreened semen for insemination) won't be "counted" as a case of woman-to-woman transmission.

Most people infected with HIV have no symptoms, since the virus can lie dormant for months and can take years to produce symptoms of AIDS. Symptoms of HIV in women resemble a number of other STDs, such as recurrent or difficult-to-treat yeast infections or PID. Use gloves on hands for finger fucking and fisting, and plastic wrap for oral sex. Cover sex toys with a condom or glove. Don't share needles, razors, or piercing/cutting instruments, and don't expose partners to your menstrual blood.

HPV (human papillomavirus). HPV is the virus commonly associated with genital and anal warts and with cervical cancer. More recently, it's been established that virtually *all* cervical cancers (99 percent) are caused by HPV, though only a few of the many strains of HPV are thought to cause cervical cancer.[20]

Woman-to-woman transmission of HPV seems certain, even among women who have never had sex with men.[21] HPV is so prevalent in the United States as to be ubiquitous, say some health educators.[22]

Like herpes, HPV can be transmitted through skin-to-skin contact when the virus is shedding—which may or may not be accompanied by the appearance of warts on the genitals or anus.

HPV can be transmitted through frottage (without clothing), hand-to-vulva, and hand-to-anus contact. You can acquire HPV by touching the affected area of a partner with your hand and then touching your own genital area without washing your hands.

Also, as with herpes, HPV can be transmitted from one mucosal membrane to another—from vulva or anus to mouth.

*I came out to my partner about being
HIV+ and having HPV on our first date.
That was one intense date, let me tell you!
We also talked about the kind of sex we like,
and we had a very hot night of sex after
our long personal discussion.*

You might discover you've been infected with HPV when warts appear on your genitals or anus. More likely, HPV is discovered through a routine Pap smear. Treatment may involve removing external genital and anal warts and treating cervical abnormalities through colposcopy, biopsy, and other procedures. HPV is infectious even after the warts are removed or cervical dysplasia disappears. There's no cure for HPV, though progression to cervical cancer can be prevented by regular gynecological screening and follow-up. Use gloves on hands for finger fucking and fisting, and plastic wrap for oral sex. Cover sex toys with a condom or glove. Change condoms and gloves between partners.

Syphilis is rarely transmitted through woman-to-woman sex—though it's possible.[23] Syphilis initially appears as a single sore or chancre. It is caused by the *treponema pallidum* bacteria and is treated with penicillin. Refrain from unprotected sex until the infection has been treated.

Trichomoniasis can be transmitted through woman-to-woman sex, through contact with vaginal secretions.[24] You can acquire trichomoniasis by touching the affected area of a partner with your hand and then touching your own genital area. Partners of an infected woman should be checked for trichomoniasis. "Trich" can lie dormant for months or years. As with bacterial vaginosis, symptoms include vaginal discharge, burning, irritation, painful urination, and strong vaginal odor. Trichomoniasis is caused by the *trichomonas vaginalis* protozoa and is treated with antibiotics. Use gloves on hands for finger fucking and fisting, and plastic wrap for oral sex. Cover sex toys with a condom or glove. Change condoms and gloves between partners.

Urinary tract infections (UTIs). While not sexually transmitted per se, urinary tract infections deserve mention because women often get UTIs when bacteria are forced into the urethra during vaginal penetration. Often women who have penetrative sex after a long hiatus get UTIs. Hence, the nickname "honeymoon disease." You'll know you have a UTI when you feel a persistent, painful need to urinate—even when your bladder is empty. If you suspect you have a UTI, see a physician immediately to prevent a more serious infection. You can help prevent UTIs by drinking a minimum of eight glasses of water a day and urinating before and after penetrative sex.

Safer Sex Is More Than Latex

The women of AABL/The Northwest Network of Bisexual, Trans and Lesbian Survivors of Abuse are quick to point out that safer sex requires more than latex—your emotional and physical safety needs must be met as well. How do you determine whether a sexual relationship is abusive? Here are some questions to ponder:

- Do you ever have sex to "keep the peace"? Or because you were tired of resisting?

- Has your partner forced you to have sex against your will?

- Has your partner refused to practice safer sex when you asked her to?

- Does your partner make fun of your sexuality? Does your partner ridicule your appearance or body size? Does she put you down or demean you during sex?

- Does your partner expect you to report to her about masturbating? Does she tell you shouldn't masturbate because it's "cheating"?

- Does your partner demand that you tell her your fantasies? Does she shame you because of your sexual desires or fantasies?

- Does your partner accuse you of having affairs? Does your partner threaten to have affairs when you both have agreed to be monogamous?

- Has your partner accused you of not being a "real" lesbian?

If you feel your relationship is abusive, get help. You can call your local (or regional) domestic violence or sexual assault hotline. Some hotlines are staffed by lesbian-friendly and transgender-friendly volunteers—after all, lesbians and bisexual women have volunteered countless hours for many local feminist antiviolence resources (and in some cases even founded them). However, be aware that not all domestic violence hotline volunteers will understand or even sympathize with the needs of lesbian, bisexual, and transgendered clients. Contact AABL to find supportive resources in your area. (See the "Resources.")

Yeast infections. According to the Lesbian-Bisexual Women's Health Study, it's unknown whether yeast infections can be transmitted sexually from woman to woman.[25] They certainly are common! Yeast infections are caused by an imbalance in normal yeast found in the vagina. It is thought that the condition can be aggravated by high sugar intake—and some woman are finding that this includes exposure to lubricants containing glycerin—by stress, or by moisture from wearing wet clothing. Symptoms include a white, clumpy vaginal discharge, and itching and burning in the vagina. Yeast infections are treated with antifungal medication. Recurrent or difficult-to-treat yeast infections may be symptomatic of diabetes, HIV, or herpes.

What If Your Partner Won't Use Barriers?

You have a right to employ safer-sex techniques—regardless of whether your partner believes STDs can or can't be transmitted through woman-to-woman sex.

Discussing safer sex is part of sexual negotiation. As with other aspects of sexual communication, you have to know what you want to tell your partner. What are your safer-sex standards? Dams for rimming? Gloves for fisting? Tell your partner.

If a woman refuses to use a barrier for oral sex, or to wear gloves for penetration, or to put a condom on her dildo, or to use lube, you don't have to have sex with her. Many women out there would love to be sexual with you *and* be respectful of your health concerns!

What If You Have an STD?

> *Sometimes I feel dirty, like nobody would want me. And when my girlfriend doesn't want to have sex with me, I immediately assume it's about my hepatitis, even though it's really about her, like she's told me a million times before. Even so, if I think about it too long I wind up beating myself up for having hep C.*

In addition to gynecological care, make sure you get emotional support, too! Acquiring an STD can wreck havoc with your self-esteem. You may feel untouchable or ashamed. Because even progressive communities at times treat STDs as moral rather than health issues, you may be left feeling as if you have no right to a sex life at all. You deserve as much pleasure now as you ever did—but you *do* have a responsibility not to transmit the STD to your partners. Practicing safer sex will prevent you from acquiring a new sexually transmitted condition, too.

Here are some things to think about and do:

- *Get treated.* Don't attempt to self-diagnose and treat your STD.

- *Follow up on gynecological care.*
- *Notify your recent sex partners,* so that they can get tested, too.
- *Care for yourself* as you would when facing any other illness. Avoid stress, eat well, get eight hours' sleep each night.
- *Don't beat yourself up.* Sexually transmitted diseases are caused by bacteria and viruses—not weak morals!
- *Take responsibility.* Don't pass the STD along to your partners. Follow recommended safer-sex guidelines (see Chapter 4, "The Road to Heaven Leads to You," and the discussion above).
- *Tell new partners about your STD.* They're responsible for their sexual health just as you are for yours. Your full disclosure enables your partners to make decisions regarding safer sex.
- In some communities, you can *find support groups* for women with herpes and other chronic STDs. If formal support structures aren't available in your area, get support from close friends or from members of Internet support groups. It helps to have someone to talk to.
- Remember: You're entitled to a fulfilling, healthy sex life. You're no less deserving of sexual pleasure because you've acquired an STD. *Play safe!*

Suggested Web Links:

LESBIANSTD.COM
   www.lesbianstd.com
SAFERSEX.ORG
   www.safersex.org/women/lesbianss.html
UNSPEAKABLE.COM
   www.unspeakable.com
STD HOME PAGE
   www.grin.net/~sycamore/std/index.html

NOTES:

1. Jeanne Marrazzo, LesbianStd.Com, www.lesbianstd.com
2. Tristan Taormino, *The Ultimate Guide to Anal Sex for Women* (Cleis Press, 1997), 123.
3. Charles Moser, Ph.D., M.D., *Health Care Without Shame: A Handbook for the Sexually Diverse and Their Caregivers* (Greenery Press, 1999), 39. www.bigrock.com/~greenery
4. Moser, *Health Care Without Shame*, 42–43.
5. LesbianSTD.com, www.lesbianstd.com
6. Patricia Kloser and Jane MacLean Craig, *The Woman's HIV Sourcebook: A Guide to Better Health and Well-Being* (Taylor Publishing, 1994), 75; Roselyn Payne Epps and Susan Cobb Stewart, eds., *The American Medical Women's Association Guide to Sexuality* (Dell Books, 1996), 158; June M. Reinisch and Ruth Beasley, *The Kinsey Institute New Report on Sex* (St. Martin's Press, 1990), 591.
7. Tristan Taormino, *The Ultimate Guide to Anal Sex for Women* (Cleis Press, 1997), XX.
8. "Nonoxy-0: May Increase HIV Risk," *Reuters Health*, reporting on the work of Dr. Roxana Rustomjee, University of Natal, South Africa, August 18, 1999.
9. Jeanne Marrazzo, conversation with the author, October 6, 1999.
10. Kathleen Stine, "Sexual Minority Women and Vulvar-Vaginal Infections," Lesbian-Bisexual Women's Health Study, University of Washington Virology Research Clinic, 1999.
11. J. Marrazzo, L. A. Koutsky, K. Stine, and S. Hillier, "Prevalence and Microbiology of Bacterial Vaginosis in Lesbians," LesbianSTD.com, www.lesbianstd.com
12. Marrazzo, conversation, October 6, 1999.
13. Stine.
14. Jeanne M. Marrazzo, Laura A. Koutsky, Kathleen L. Stine, et al., "Genital Human Papillomavirus in Women Who Have Sex with Women," *Journal of Infectious Diseases*, vol. 178, 1604–609, 1998. Marrazzo found that of the 149 women, 147 had digital-vaginal sex with women in the prior year. The same number had cunnilingus in the prior year. More than half used insertive sex toys in the prior year. More than half had anal sex with women in the prior year. Slightly more than a third had engaged in rimming in the prior year.
15. Marrazzo, conversation, October 6, 1999.
16. Ibid.
17. Unspeakable.com, www.unspeakable.com/facts/chlamydia.html
18. C. Everett Koop, www.epidemic.org
19. *The American Medical Women's Association Guide to Sexuality*, Roselyn Payne Epps and Susan Cobb Stewart, eds. (New York: Dell Books, 1996), 140.
20. "Human Papillomavirus Is a Necessary Cause of Invasive Cervical Cancer Worldwide," by Jan M. M. Walboomers, Marcel V. Jacobs, M. Michele Manos, et al., *Journal of Pathology*, vol. 189, issue 1.
21. Marrazzo, Koutsky, Stine, et al., "Genital Human Papillomavirus," 1604-609.
22. Stine.
23. Ibid.
24. Marrazzo, conversation, October 6, 1999.
25. Stine.

SOURCE OF SIDEBARS:

LesbianSTD.com, excerpted with permission from www.lesbianstd.com

"Safer Sex Is More Than Just Latex" reprinted from a flier, with permission, of AABL/The Northwest Network of Bisexual, Trans and Lesbian Survivors of Abuse.

chapter seventeen

Bibliography

Articles

"Anatomical Relationship Between Urethra and
Clitoris," by Helen E. O'Connell, John M.
Huston, Colin R. Anderson, and Robert J.
Plenter. *Journal of Urology*, vol. 159, 1892–97,
June 1990.

"Aphrodite's Appetite: The Ins and Outs of Eating
for Great Sex," by Heather Corinna. *Scarlet
Letters: A Journal of Femmerotica*, May 1999.

"Between Women: Activists Hope for Answers
from the First Federal Study of Lesbian
Transmission of HIV," by Sue Rochman. *The
Advocate*, May 25, 1999, 73–74.

"Cervical Cancer Risk and Papanicolaou Screening
in a Sample of Lesbian and Bisexual Women," by
Elizabeth J. Rankow and Irene Tessaro. *Journal of
Family Practice*, vol. 47, no. 2, 139–43, August
1998.

"Female Ejaculation: Perceived Origins, the
Grafenberg Spot/Area, and Sexual Responsive-
ness," by Carol Ann Darling, J. Kenneth Davidson,
Sr., and Colleen Conway-Welch. *Archives of
Sexual Behavior*, vol. 19, no. 1, 29–47, 1990.

"Genital Human Papillomavirus Infection in
Women Who Have Sex with Women," by
Jeanne M. Marrazzo, Laura A. Koutsky, Kathleen
L. Strine, et al. *Journal of Infectious Diseases*, vol.
178, 1604–609, 1999.

"Health Related Behaviors and Cancer Screening
of Lesbians: Results from the Boston Lesbian
Health Project," by Susan Jo Roberts and Lena
Sorensen. *Women and Health*, vol. 28, no. 4,
1–11, 1999.

"Human Papillomavirus Infection: The Most
Common Sexually Transmitted Infection," by
Kathleen Stine. *Journal of the Gay and Lesbian
Medical Association*, vol. 3, no. 1, 21–22, 1999.

"Optimal Gynecologic and Obstetric Care for
Lesbians," by Nina M. Carroll. *Obstetrics and
Gynecology*, vol. 93, no. 4, 611–13, April 1999.

Audiotapes and CD-ROMs

The audiotapes and CD-ROMs listed below are
available from Passion Press, P.O. Box 277,
Newark, CA 94560.
Tel. (800) 724 3284
Fax (510) 644.1945
www.passionpress.com
info@passionpress.com

"Cyborgasm" and "Cyborgasm 2"
Produced by Lisa Palac
Recorded with virtual reality technology for a
3D sound. "Cyborgasm" features Annie Sprinkle,
Susie Bright, and Mistress Kat; "Cyborgasm 2"
features Susie Bright, Lisa Palac, and Carol
Queen. (Headphones required for 3-D sound.)
Available on cassette and CD.
60 min. each.

"Herotica," "Herotica 2," "Herotica 3," "Herotica 4"
Available on cassette and CD.
180 min. each.

Books

BISEXUALITY

Bi Any Other Name: Bisexual People Speak Out,
edited by Loraine Hutchins and Lani
Kaahumanu (Alyson Publications, 1991).

Bisexual Resource Guide 2000, edited by Robyn
Ochs (Bisexual Resource Center, 1999).

*Real Live Nude Girl: Chronicles of Sex-Positive
Culture*, by Carol Queen (Cleis Press, 1997).

*Vice Versa: Bisexuality and the Eroticism of Everyday
Life*, by Marjorie B. Garber (Simon & Schuster,
1996).

EROTICA

Afterglow: More Stories of Lesbian Desire, edited by
Karen Barber (Alyson Publications, 1993).

Best Lesbian Erotica 2000, selected and introduced by Joan Nestle, Tristan Taormino series editor (Cleis Press, 2000).

Best Lesbian Erotica 1999, selected and introduced by Chrystos, Tristan Taormino series editor (Cleis Press, 1999).

Best Lesbian Erotica 1998, selected and introduced by Jewelle Gomez, Tristan Taormino series editor (Cleis Press, 1998).

Black Feathers: Erotic Dreams, by Cecilia Tan (HarperCollins, 1998).

Dark Angels: Lesbian Vampire Stories, edited by Pam Keesey (Cleis Press, 1994).

Daughters of Darkness: Lesbian Vampire Stories, edited by Pam Keesey (Cleis Press, 1993).

Doc and Fluff: The Dystopian Tale of a Girl and Her Biker, by Pat Califia (Alyson Publications, 1996).

Doing It for Daddy: Short Sexy Fiction About a Very Forbidden Fantasy, edited by Pat Califia (Alyson Publications, 1994).

Friday the Rabbi Wore Lace: Jewish Lesbian Erotica, edited by Karen X. Tulchinsky (Cleis Press, 1998).

Heatwave Women in Love and Lust: Lesbian Short Fiction, edited by Lucy Jane Bledsoe (Alyson Publications, 1995).

Hot and Bothered: Short Fiction of Lesbian Desire, edited by Karen X. Tulchinsky (Arsenal Pulp, 1998).

The Leather Daddy and the Femme: An Erotic Novel, by Carol Queen (Cleis Press, 1998).

Leatherwomen III: The Clash of the Cultures, edited by Laura Antoniou (Masquerade Books, 1998).

Macho Sluts, by Pat Califia (Alyson Publications, 1989).

Melting Point, by Pat Califia (Alyson Publications, 1996).

Pillow Talk: Lesbian Stories Between the Covers, edited by Lesléa Newman (Alyson Publications, 1998).

Speaking in Whispers: Lesbian African-American Erotica, by Kathleen E. Morris (Third Side Press, 1996).

Switch Hitters: Lesbians Write Gay Male Erotica and Gay Men Write Lesbian Erotica, edited by Carol Queen and Lawrence Schimel (Cleis Press, 1997).

Virgin Territory and *Virgin Territory 2*, edited by Shar Rednour (Masquerade Books, 1996, 1997).

GENDER

Body Alchemy: Transsexual Portraits, by Loren Cameron (Cleis Press, 1996).

Butch/Femme: Inside Lesbian Gender, by Sally R. Munt and Cherry Smith (Cassell, 1998).

Dagger: On Butch Women, edited by Roxxie, Lily Burana, and Linnea Due (Cleis Press, 1994).

Drag King Book: A First Look, by Del LaGrace Volcano and Judith "Jack" Halberstam (Serpent's Tail, 1999).

Female Masculinity, by Judith Halberstam (Duke University Press, 1998).

Femme: Feminists, Lesbians, and Bad Girls, edited by Laura Harris and Elizabeth Crocker (Routledge, 1997).

The Femme's Guide to the Universe, by Shar Rednour (Alyson Publications, 2000).

The Femme Mystique, by Lesléa Newman (Alyson Publications, 1995).

FTM: Female-to-Male Transsexuals in Society, by Holly Devor (Indiana University Press, 1997).

Gender Outlaw: On Men, Women, and the Rest of Us, by Kate Bornstein (Vintage, 1995).

Intersex in the Age of Ethics, edited by Alice Domurat Dreger (University Press Group, 1999).

The Last Time I Wore a Dress, by Daphne Scholinski and Jane Meredith Adams (Putnam, 1997).

Lesbians Talk Transgender, by Zachary I. Nataf (Scarlet Press, 1996).

My Gender Workbook, by Kate Bornstein (Routledge, 1998).

The Persistent Desire: A Femme–Butch Reader, edited by Joan Nestle (Alyson Publications, 1992).

Read My Lips: Sexual Subversion and the End of Gender, by Riki Anne Wilchins (Firebrand Books, 1997).

Sex Changes: The Politics of Transgenderism, by Pat Califia (Cleis Press, 1997).

Transgender Care: Recommended Guidelines, Practical Information, and Personal Accounts, by Gianna E. Israel, Donald E. Tarver, and Joy Diane Shaffer (Temple University Press, 1997).

Transgender Warriors: Making History from Joan of Arc to Dennis Rodman, by Leslie Feinberg (Beacon, 1997).

Trans Liberation: Beyond Pink or Blue, by Leslie Feinberg (Beacon, 1998).

Transmen and FTMs: Identities, Bodies, Genders, and Sexualities, by Jason Cromwell (University of Illinois Press, 1999).

ORGASM

Becoming Orgasmic: A Sexual and Personal Growth Program for Women, by Julia R. Heiman, Ph.D., and Joseph Lopiccolo, Ph.D. (Fireside/Simon & Schuster, 1988).

Camino al Orgasmo, by Sonia Blasco (Simon & Schuster, 1993).

For Yourself: The Fulfillment of Female Sexuality, by Lonnie Barbach, Ph.D. (Signet/Penguin, 1975).

When the Earth Moves: Women and Orgasm, by Mikaya Heart (Celestial Arts, 1998).

PHOTOGRAPHY

Body Alchemy: Transsexual Portraits, by Loren Cameron (Cleis Press, 1996).

Butch/Femme, edited by M. G. Soares (Crown, 1995).

Drag King Book: A First Look, by Del LaGrace Volcano and Judith "Jack" Halberstam (Serpent's Tail, 1999).

Femalia, edited by Joani Blank (Down There Press, 1993).

Her Tongue on My Theory: Images, Essays, and Fantasies, by Kiss and Tell (Press Gang Publishers, 1994).

I Am My Lover: Women Pleasure Themselves, edited by Joani Blank (Down There Press, 1997).

Nothing but the Girl: The Blatant Lesbian Image, by Susie Bright and Jill Posner (Cassell, 1996).

RELATIONSHIPS

Allies in Healing: When the Person You Love Was Sexually Abused as a Child: A Support Book, by Laura Davis (HarperPerennial, 1991).

The Ethical Slut: A Guide to Infinite Sexual Possibilities, by Dossie Easton and Catherine Liszt (Greenery Press, 1998).

Feathering Your Nest: An Interactive Guide to a Loving Lesbian Relationship, by Gwen Leonhard and Jennie Mast (Rising Tide, 1996).

The Intimacy Dance: A Guide to Long-Term Success in Gay and Lesbian Relationships, by Betty Berzon (Plume, 1997).

The Lesbian and Gay Book of Love and Marriage: Creating the Stories of Our Lives, by Paula Martinac (Broadway Books, 1998).

Lesbian Couples: Creating Healthy Relationships for the '90s, by D. Merilee Clunis (Seal Press, 1993).

The Lesbian Couples' Guide: Finding the Right Woman and Creating a Life Together, by Judith McDaniel (HarperPerennial, 1995).

The Lesbian Love Companion: How to Survive Everything from Heartthrob to Heartbreak, by Marny Hall (HarperSanFrancisco, 1998).

Lesbian Polyfidelity, by Celeste West (Booklegger Press, 1995).

Staying Power: Long-Term Lesbian Couples, by Susan E. Johnson (Naiad, 1990).

SEX GUIDES AND HOW-TO

Anal Pleasure and Health: A Guide for Men and Women, by Jack Morin (Down There Press, 1998).

Are We Having Fun Yet? The Intelligent Woman's Guide to Sex, by Marcia Douglass, Ph.D., and Lisa Douglass, Ph.D. (Hyperion, 1997).

Big Big Love: A Sourcebook on Sex for People of Size and Those Who Love Them, by Hanne Blank (Greenery Press, 1999).

The Black Book, 5th ed., by Bill Brent (Black Books, 1998).

The Erotic Mind: Unlocking the Inner Sources of Sexual Passion and Fulfillment, by Jack Morin (HarperPerennial, 1996).

Exhibitionism for the Shy, by Carol Queen (Down There Press, 1995).

First Person Sexual: Women and Men Write About Self-Pleasuring, edited by Joani Blank (Down There Press, 1996).

The Good Vibrations Guide to Adult Videos, by Cathy Winks (Down There Press, 1998).

The Good Vibrations Guide to the G-Spot, by Cathy Winks (Down There Press, 1998).

Good Vibrations: The Complete Guide to Vibrators, by Joani Blank (Down There Press, 1989).

A Hand in the Bush: The Art of Vaginal Fisting, by Deborah Addington (Greenery Press, 1996).

Lesbian Passion: Loving Ourselves and Each Other, by Joann Loulan (Spinsters, 1987).

Lesbian Sex, by Joann Loulan (Spinsters, 1984).

The Lesbian Sex Book, by Wendy Caster (Alyson Publications, 1993).

The New Good Vibrations Guide to Sex, by Cathy Winks and Anne Semans (Cleis Press, 1997).

"Safer Sex Handbook for Lesbians," by Cynthia Madansky and Julie Tolentino Wood (GMHC, 1993, pamphlet).

Sapphistry: The Book of Lesbian Sexuality, by Pat Califia (Naiad Press, 1979).

Sex for One: The Joy of Selfloving, by Betty Dodson (Crown, 1996).

The Sexuality of Latinas, edited by Norma Alarcon, Ana Castillo, and Cherrie Moraga (Third Woman Press, 1993). In English and Spanish.

The Strap-on Book, by A. H. Dion (Greenery Press, 1999).

The Survivor's Guide to Sex: How to Have an Empowered Sex Life After Child Sexual Abuse, by Staci Haines (Cleis Press, 1999).

Susie Sexpert's Lesbian Sex World, by Susie Bright (Cleis Press, 1990, 1998).

The Ultimate Guide to Anal Sex for Women, by Tristan Taormino (Cleis Press, 1997).

The Ultimate Guide to Strap-on Sex: A Resource for Men and Women, by Karlyn Lotney (Cleis Press, 1999).

The Woman's Guide to Sex on the Web, by Anne Semans and Cathy Winks (HarperSanFrancisco, 1999).

SEXUAL POLITICS

Annie Sprinkle's Post-Porn Modernist: My 25 Years as a Multimedia Whore, by Annie Sprinkle (Cleis Press, 1997).

Caught Looking: Feminism, Pornography, and Censorship, edited by the FACT Book Committee (LongRiver Books, 1986).

Her Tongue on My Theory: Images, Essays, and Fantasies, by Kiss and Tell (Press Gang Publishers, 1994).

I Used to Be Nice: Reflections on Feminist and Lesbian Politics, by Sue O'Sullivan (Cassell, 1996).

PoMoSexuals: Challenging Assumptions about Gender and Identity, edited by Carol Queen and Lawrence Schimel (Cleis Press, 1997).

Public Sex: The Culture of Radical Sex, by Pat Califia (Cleis Press, 1994).

Sex Work: Writings by Women in the Sex Industry, edited by Frédérique Delacoste and Priscilla Alexander (Cleis Press, 1987, 1998).

Technology of Orgasm: "Hysteria," the Vibrator, and Women's Sexual Satisfaction, by Rachel P. Maines (Johns Hopkins University Press, 1999).

S/M AND FETISH SEX

Blood Bound: Guidance for the Responsible Vampyre, by Deborah Addington and Vincent Dior (Greenery Press, 1999).

The Bottoming Book: How to Get Terrible Things Done to You by Wonderful People, by Dossie Easton and Catherine A. Liszt (Greenery Press, 1998).

Coming to Power: Writings and Graphics on Lesbian S/M, 3d ed., edited by SAMOIS (Alyson Publications, 1987).

The Compleat Spanker, by Lady Green (Greenery Press, 1998).

Juice: Electricity for Pleasure and Pain, by Uncle Abdul (Greenery Press, 1998).

Kinkycrafts: 99 Do-It-Yourself S/M Toys for the Kinky Handyperson, edited by Lady Green (Greenery Press, 1998).

The Lesbian S/M Safety Manual, edited by Pat Califia (Alyson Publications, 1988).

The Second Coming: A Leatherdyke Reader, edited by Pat Califia and Robin Sweeney (Alyson Publications, 1996).

The Sexually Dominant Woman: A Workbook for Nervous Beginners, by Lady Green (Greenery Press, 1998).

The Topping Book: Or, Getting Good at Being Bad, by Dossie Easton and Catherine A. Liszt (Greenery Press, 1998).

SPIRITUALITY AND SEX

The Art of Sexual Ecstasy: The Path of Sacred Sexuality for Western Lovers, by Margo Anand (Tarcher, 1991).

Bitch Goddess: The Spiritual Path of the Dominant Woman, edited by Pat Califia and Drew Campbell (Greenery Press, 1988).

Lesbian Sacred Sexuality, by Diane Mariechild and Marcelina Martin (Wingbow Press, 1995).

Sacred Sex, by Jwala (Mandala, 1993).

WOMEN'S BODIES AND HEALTH

The Black Women's Health Book, edited by Evelyn C. White (Seal Press, 1994).

Bridging the Gap: A National Directory of Services for Women and Girls with Disabilities, 2d ed., by Ellen Rubin, edited by Merle Froschl (Educational Equity Concepts, Inc., 1998).

Cunt: A Declaration of Independence, by Inga Muscio (Seal Press, 1998).

Dating Violence: Young Women in Danger, edited by Barrie Levy (Seal Press, 1998).

Dr. Susan Love's Breast Book, by Susan M. Love and Karen Lindsey (Perseus, 1995).

Dr. Susan Love's Hormone Book: Making Informed Choices About Menopause, by Susan M. Love and Karen Lindsey (Random House, 1998).

Femalia, edited by Joani Blank (Down There Press, 1993).

Getting Free: You Can End Abuse and Take Back Your Life, by Ginny NiCarthy (Seal Press, 1997).

Good for You: A Handbook on Lesbian Health and Wellbeing, by Tamsin Wilton (Cassell, 1999).

Health Care Without Shame: A Handbook for the Sexually Diverse and Their Caregivers, by Charles Moser, Ph.D., M.D. (Greenery Press, 1999).

The Lesbian Health Book: Caring for Ourselves, edited by Marissa C. Martinez and Jocelyn C. White (Seal Press, 1997).

The New Ourselves, Growing Older: Women Aging with Knowledge and Power, by Paula B. Doress-Worters and Diana Laskin Siegal (Touchstone/Simon & Schuster, 1994).

A New View of a Woman's Body, by the Federation of Feminist Women's Health Centers (Feminist Health Press, 1991).

Off the Rag: Lesbians Writing on Menopause, edited by Lee Lynch and Akia Woods (New Victoria Press, 1996).

Our Bodies, Ourselves: For the New Century, by the Boston Women's Health Book Collective (Touchstone/Simon & Schuster, 1998).

Parting Company: Understanding the Loss of a Loved One: The Caregiver's Journey, by Cynthia Pearson and Margaret L. Stubbs (Seal Press, 1999).

Restricted Access: Lesbians on Disability, edited by Victoria A. Brownworth and Susan Raffo (Seal Press, 1999).

The Ultimate Guide to Pregnancy for Lesbians: Tips and Techniques from Conception to Birth—How to Stay Sane and Care for Yourself, by Rachel Pepper (Cleis Press, 1999).

The Vagina Monologues, by Eve Ensler (Villard, 1998).

Women En Large: Images of Fat Nudes, by Laurie Edison and Debbie Notkin (Books in Focus, 1994).

You Don't Have to Take It!: A Woman's Guide to Confronting Emotional Abuse at Work, by Ginny NiCarthy, Naomi Gottlieb, and Sandra Coffman (Seal Press, 1993).

E-Zines

Body Modification E-Zine
Electronic magazine devoted to all forms of body modification (from tattoos to genital piercing to surgical modifications). Contains photo galleries, articles, interviews, personal ads, and chat. Earn a free membership by submitting a photo or an article about your own body modification experiences. 247 Bathurst St., Toronto, ON, M5T 2S4, Canada
www.bmezine.com
shannon@bmezine.com

Dentata
"A Magazine for Chicks with the Package." A new magazine that intends to give voice to HIV-positive women, as well as both men and women who are sexually involved with HIV-positive women, and to provide fun, open, and lively discussion on all matters sexual. P.O. Box 3214, Hollywood, CA 90078
www.chickpages.com/zinescene/dentata/index.html
DentataMag@aol.com

Electric Edge
Free online edition of *Ragged Edge,* the magazine on disability (formerly *Disability Rag*). Features "the best in today's writing about society's 'ragged edge' issues: medical rationing, genetic discrimination, assisted suicide, long-term care, attendant services."
www.ragged-edge-mag.com

FLASH—The Deaf Queer E-Zine
A free electronic 'zine published by CTN, a national magazine for deaf lesbians, gays, and bisexuals.
www.deafqueer.org/ctnmagazine/FLASH/index.html

KUMA
Black lesbian erotica.
members.tripod.com/~Versai/title.htm

Nerve
Literate smut.
www.nerve.com/

Roughriders
The erotic fiction e-zine for FTMs of all sexual persuasions.
www.netgsi.com/~transman/roughriders.html

Scarlet Letters: A Journal of Femmerotica
Erotica web-zine.
P.O. Box 60855, Chicago, IL 60660
www.scarletletters.com
scarletletters@yahoo.com

Sistah Scape Online
Monthly web magazine dedicated to issues
affecting lesbian women of color.
www.sistahscape.com/about.html

Magazines

Anything That Moves
Bisexual quarterly features stories, poetry, news.
2261 Market St., Ste. 496, San Francisco, CA 94114
(415) 626-5069
www.anythingthatmoves.com
info@anythingthatmoves.com

Bad Attitude
Lesbian S/M fiction.
P.O. Box 39110, Cambridge, MA 02139

Bitch
Feminist response to pop culture—"a print
magazine devoted to incisive commentary on our
media-driven world."
3128 16th Street, P.O. Box 143,
San Francisco, CA 94103
(415) 864-6671
www.bitchmagazine.com
lisa@bitchmagazine.com

Black Sheets
Pansexual 'zine.
www.queernet.org/BlackBooks

Bust
"*Bust* is the magazine of choice for today's sassy
girls who know that *Vogue* is vapid, *Glamour* is
garbage, and *Cosmo* is clueless. Fierce, funny, and
too smart to be anything but feminist, *Bust* is the
voice of the new girl order."
www.bust.com
bust@aol.com

Curve Magazine
2336 Market Street, Ste. 5, San Francisco, CA
94114
(415) 863-6538
Fax (415) 863-1609

Diva
The U.K.'s lesbian magazine.
116–134, Bayham St., London, England NW1 0BA
www.gaytimes.co.uk
diva@gaytimes.co.uk

Dykes, Disability, and Stuff
An aggressive proponent of greater access to
lesbian culture and community. All
advertisements and notices accepted for
publication must provide information on the
forms of access provided. If you are a lesbian
with a disability or a lesbian wanting to inform
yourself about disability issues, write for a four-
issue subscription.
Available in standard print, large print,
audiocassette, braille, DOS disk, or modem
transfer.
P.O. Box 8773, Madison, WI 53708
tps.stdorg.wisc.edu/MGLRC/Groups/DykesDisabi
litiesStuff.html

Fabula Magazine
For the female mind.
55 Norfolk St., Ste. 202, San Francisco, CA 94103
(415) 255-8926
www.fabulamag.com
fabula@vdn.com

Fat!So?
For people who don't apologize for their size.
P.O. Box 423464, San Francisco, CA 94142
marilyn@fatso.com

Girlfriends
The Magazine of Lesbian Culture, Politics, and
Entertainment
HAF Enterprises
3415 Cesar Chavez, Suite 101
San Francisco, CA 94110
(415) 648-9464
Fax: (415) 648-4705
www.gfriends.com

Hues

Hues stands for "Hear Us Emerging Sisters," the multicultural magazine for young women.
P.O. Box 3620, Duluth, MN 55803
(800) HUES-4U2
www.hues.net
hues@hues.net

Lesbians On the Loose

Australia's leading lesbian magazine. Monthly.
P.O. Box 1099, Darlinghurst, Australia 1300
Fax + 61 2 9380 6529
www.lotl.com
lotl@lotl.com

Lespress

Germany's magazine for lesbian and forward-thinking women. Published monthly since 1995; circulation 10,000. Interviews/profiles, erotica, events calendar, lesmopolitan (news and stories from around the world), and reviews of CDs, films, and books.
Kaiser-Karl-Ring 57, D-53111 Bonn
Tel. +49 (0)228 653464
Fax +49 (0)228 653501
www.lespress.de
info@lespress.de

On Our Backs

The Best of Lesbian Sex
HAF Enterprises
3415 César Chavez, Ste. 101,
San Francisco, CA 94110
Tel. (415) 648-9464
Fax (415) 648-4705
www.gfriends.com/onourbacks
staff@gfriends.con

Skin Two

The world's leading fetish art, fashion, nightlife, and newsmagazine. *Skin Two* online is a comprehensive interactive fetish web site. Membership fee.
Unit 63, Abbey Business Centre, Ingate Place, London SW8 3NS
Tel. +44 (0) 171 498 5533
Fax +44 (0) 171 498 5565
www.skintwo.co.uk
online@skintwo.co.uk

Transgender Tapestry Magazine

Quarterly magazine "by, for, and about all things trans, including cross-dressing, transsexualism, intersexuality, FTM, MTF, butch, femme, drag kings and drag queens, androgyny, female and male impersonation, and more."
IFGE, P.O. Box 540229, Waltham, MA 02545
www.ifge.org/tgmag/tgmagtop.htm
editor@ifge.org

Transsexual News Telegraph (TNT)

Transsexual /transgendered-focused magazine.
41 Sutter St., Ste. 1124, San Francisco, CA 94104
(415) 703-7161 (leave message), (415) 775-3848
GailTNT@aol.com

Zaftig!

Sex for the well rounded.
54 Boynton St., 1st Floor, Boston, MA 02130
www.xensei.com/users/zaftig/home.htm
zaftig@xensei.com

Videos

Hundreds of porn videos feature girl-on-girl sex.
This list emphasizes woman-produced and lesbian-
produced videos. Where to find videos? You can
purchase them from many of the mail-order and
retail outlets in these resource listings and from the
producers (listed below). You can rent videos from
The Blue Door.

VIDEO SOURCES:

Annie Sprinkle's videos may be ordered from
Gates of Heck
(800) 213-8170
www.heck.com
sprinkle@heck.com

Betty Dodson's videos may be ordered from Betty
Dodson Productions
P.O. Box 1933, Murray Hill, New York, NY
10156
www.bettydodson.com
site@bettydodson.com

Bleu Visions
Bleu Productions, Inc.
P.O. Box 20280, New York, NY 10011
www.bleuproductions.com
info@bleuproductions.com

Fatale Video
1537 4th Street, Ste. 193, San Rafael, CA 94901
(888) 5-FATALE
www.other-rooms.com/fatale.html
fatale@other-rooms.com

Femme Productions
www.royalle.com

House O' Chicks
2215R Market St., Ste. 813, San Francisco, CA
94114
Tel. (415) 861-9849
Fax (415) 626 5049
www.houseochicks.com
dorrie@houseochicks.com

EROTICA

"The Black Glove"
  Bleu Visions. Maria Beatty. 1996 30 min.

"The Boiler Room"
  Bleu Visions. Maria Beatty. 1998 51 min.

"Burlezk Live!" and "Burlezk II Live!"
  Fatale Videos.

"Clips"
  Fatale Video. Three ten-minute lesbian-smut
  vignettes, including Fanny Fatale's famous
  ejaculation scene. 1988 30 min.

"Dress Up for Daddy"
  Fatale Videos. Real-life lesbian lovers do Daddy
  play.

"The Elegant Spanking"
  Bleu Visions. Maria Beatty and Rosemary Delain.
  1995 30 min.

"Hungry Hearts"
  Fatale Videos. Real-life lovers Pepper and
  Reeva. 30 min.

"Leda and the Swan—Nailed"
  Bleu Visions. Maria Beatty. 1999 42 min.

"Private Pleasures"
  Fatale Videos. Butch/femme sex and fisting.
  1985 30 min.

"Safe Is Desire"
  Fatale Videos. Take a trip to a lesbian sex club.

"San Francisco Lesbians," vol. 1–8
  Pleasure. Not only are these real lesbians having
  real sex—but they also feature a wide range of
  sexual styles. 1992–1994 85 min.

"Sassy Schoolgirl"
  Bleu Visions. Maria Beatty. 1998 45 min.

"Shadows"
  Fatale Videos. Lesbian S/M dungeon scene.
  1985 30 min.

"She's Safe"
Frameline Arts Foundation. If you think safe sex is, well, dry, check out this compilation of lesbian-made shorts. 1993 40 min.

"Suburban Dykes"
Fatale Videos. Nina Hartley and Sharon Mitchel. 1990 30 min.

Sex Guides and How-To

"Annie Sprinkle's Herstory of Porn"
Directed by Annie Sprinkle and Scarlot Harlot. Annie Sprinkle's film diary of 25 years of making porn. Based on the stage show directed by Emilio Cubeiro. 1998 69 min.

"Bend Over, Boyfriend"
Fatale Video. Directed by Shar Rednour. Sex-ed goddess Carol Queen and friends. 1998 60 min.

"Bend Over, Boyfriend 2: More Rockin', Less Talkin'"
Fatale Video. Directed by Shar Rednour. Sex-ed goddess Carol Queen and friends. 1999 60 min.

"Carol Queen's Great Vibrations"
Joani Blank. Carol Queen shows you everything you need to know about vibrators. 1995 55 min.

"Celebrating Orgasm"
Betty Dodson. Betty Dodson demonstrates her masturbation coaching techniques in private sessions with five different women. 1996 60 min.

"Faces of Ecstasy"
Joani Blank. Ten women and three men of diverse ages, sizes, and races masturbate to orgasm for the camera. 55 min.

"Fire in the Valley"
Annie Sprinkle and Joseph Kramer How-to workshop on female genital massage. 1999 55 min.

"How to Female Ejaculate"
Fatale Videos. Remember that hot ejaculation scene in "Clips"? Now Fanny Fatale shares her skill with a group of women whom she teaches to squirt. 1992 47 min.

"How to Find Your Goddess Spot"
House O' Chicks. Dorrie Lane teaches in G-spot play. Features the Wondrous Vulva Puppet.

"Linda/Les and Annie: The First Female to Male Transsexual Love Story"
Annie Sprinkle. Annie's video documentary of her relationship with her FTM lover. 1990 32 min.

"Magic of Female Ejaculation"
House O' Chicks. Dorrie Lane shares her own experience of female ejaculation in House O' Chicks' most popular video.

"Masturbation Memoirs 1 and 2"
House O' Chicks
Directed by Carol Leigh (aka Scarlot Harlot) Dorrie Lane sought out sex experts—women in their 40s and 50s who could share their experiences of masturbation. Annie Sprinkle, Juliet Carr, Scarlot Harlot, and Anna Marti.

"Masturbation Memoirs 3 and 4"
House O' Chicks. "...the voice and sexual expression of young, multi-cultural Lesbians."

"Nina Hartley's Guide to Anal Sex"
Porn star and sex-positive activist Nina Hartley proves to be a great teacher, too! 1996 60 min.

"Nina Hartley's Guide to Cunnilingus"
Porn star and sex-positive activist Nina Hartley proves to be a great teacher, too! 1994 45 min.

"Selfloving"
Betty Dodson's women's masturbation workshop featuring ten women, ages 28 to 60, exploring their sexuality. 1991 60 min.

"The Sluts and Goddesses Video Workshop: Or How to Be a Sex Goddess in 101 Easy Steps"
Annie Sprinkle and Maria Beatty. 1992 52 min.

"Ultimate Guide to Anal Sex for Women"
Tristan Taormino, Ernest Greene, and John
Stagliano. Based on Tristan Taormino's popular
book. Taormino leads an all-star coed cast in a
sexy anal sex workshop. Two volumes. If you liked
the book, you'll love the movie. 1999 210 min.

"Viva la Vulva"
Betty Dodson's close-up on female genital
anatomy with ten women posing for their pussy
portraits. 1998 51 min.

"Zen Pussy: A Stimulating Meditation
on Eleven Vulvas"
Annie Sprinkle and Joseph Kramer. 1999
60 min.

chapter eighteen

Resources

Bisexuality Resources

BiFems
Web ring intended to increase the visibility of
bisexual women. Links to dozens of personal
home pages.
www.lunamorena.net/BiFem
darkmoon@calweb.com

Bisexual Resource Center
Educational and support center. Publishes the
Bisexual Resource Guide, facilitates Boston-area
support groups for people who are or think they
might be bisexual, houses the bisexual archives,
and organizes conferences. Web site features
resources and links.
P.O. Box 400639, Cambridge, MA 02140
(617) 424-9595
www.biresource.org
brc@biresource.org

Disability Resources

Deaf Lesbian Resources
www.deafwoman.com/deaflesbian

The Deaf Queer Resource Center
A national nonprofit resource and information
center. Web site features links to chat rooms,
bulletin boards, mailing lists, and more.
www.deafqueer.org
www.deafqueer.org/411/faq.html
feedback@deafqueer.org

DisAbled Women's Network (DAWN)
Ontario's province-wide organization for women
with all types of disabilities. DAWN is a feminist
organization that supports women in their
struggles to control their own lives. Web site
includes an annotated bibliography about
violence against women with disabilities.
www.dawn.tyenet.com

Educational Equity Concepts, Inc.
Promotes bias-free learning through research
programs and publications. Specifically publishes
resources for women and girls with disabilities.
114 East 32nd St., New York, NY 10016
Voice/TTY (212) 725-1803
Fax (212) 725-0947
www.edequity.org
information@edequity.org

GimpGirl Community
Created by a group of young women with
disabilities, from varying backgrounds, who faced
a huge lack of support services for themselves
and others like them. "We strive to enlighten,
empower and support young women of all colors,
creeds, and sexual preferences." Feature articles,
opinion surveys, newsletter, mailing lists, and
links.
c/o The Center for Breaking Away
P.O. Box 379, Santa Cruz, CA 95061
Tel. (831) 427-5529
Fax (831) 426-8160
www.gimpgirl.com
ggc@gimpgirl.com

"Sexuality and Disability: An Annotated
Bibliography"
SIECUS (Sexuality Information and Education
Council of the United States)
www.siecus.org/pubs/biblio/bibs0009.html
siecus@siecus.org

Gender and Intersex Resources

American Boyz

Serves people who were labeled female at birth but who feel that is not an accurate or complete description of who they are, such as tomboys, butches, cross-dressers, drag kings, genderbenders, transsexuals, transgenderists, intersexuals, and other gender-variant people, along with their significant others, friends, families, and allies. The organization hosts an annual national conference and publishes a newsletter. American Boyz has affiliates throughout North America.
National Office:

212-A So. Bridge St., Ste. 131,
Elkton, MD 21921
Tel. (410) 392-3640
Fax (410) 620-2024
www.netgsi.com/~amboyz/index.html
amboyz@iximd.com

FTM Informational Network

The FTM International Network web site is packed with information—legal and political news, sources for testosterone, packin' gear in several sizes, personal stories, shaving tips, and clothing advice.
www.thegrid.net/ftminfnet
jmccracken@thegrid.net

FTM International, Inc.

FTM International represents a diverse group of transgendered men: "We come from different backgrounds, include every imaginable sexual orientation, and are multi-cultural. We are at various points along the transgender-transsexual continuum. Some of us have entered transition, beginning with self-exploration with peers or with counselors. Many of us take hormones or have surgery. Others, while having a male gender identity, believe hormones and surgery are not necessary to actualize their masculinity." Holds meetings in the San Francisco Bay Area, helps organize conferences, and publishes a newsletter.
1360 Mission St., Ste. 200,
San Francisco, CA 94103
(415) 553-5987 [voice-mail]
www.ftm-intl.org
TSTGMen@aol.com

IFGE

The International Foundation for Gender Education, founded in 1978, aspires to be the "leading advocate and educational organization for promoting self-definition and free expression of individual gender identity." Also publishes *Transgender Tapestry.*
P.O. Box 540229, Waltham, MA 02254
Tel. (781) 899-2212
Fax (781) 899-5703
www.ifge.org
info@ifge.org

Intersex Society of North America (ISNA)

A peer support, education, and advocacy group founded and operated by and for intersexuals: individuals born with anatomy or physiology that differs from cultural ideals of male and female. Publishes a newsletter, *Hermaphrodites with Attitude* and maintains web site.
P.O. Box 3070, Ann Arbor, MI 48106
www.isna.org
info@isna.org

Press for Change

A political lobbying and educational organization working to achieve equality and respect for all transsexual and transgender people in the United Kingdom. The well-written web site reads like a London *Times* of the trans world.
www.pfc.org.uk
editor@pfc.org.uk

SOFFA

SOFFA provides support for significant others, families, friends, and allies of transgendered persons.
members.aol.com/SOFFAUSA/index.html
soffausa@aol.com

Transexual Menace International

Activist organization with chapters in New York; Boston; Portland, Oregon; and Atlanta.
www.apocalypse.org/pub/tsmenace

Health Resources

AABL/The Northwest Network of Lesbian
Bisexual and Trans Survivors of Abuse
  Formerly called Advocates for Abused and
  Battered Lesbians (AABL). Provides counseling,
  support, legal advocacy, and peer support groups
  to lesbian, bisexual, and trans folks who have
  been emotionally, psychologically, physically, or
  sexually abused by their intimate partners. Also
  provides community education, training, and
  consultation about battering/abuse and
  homophobia. Leather friendly, wheelchair
  accessible. Web site features directory of local
  resources throughout the United States, Canada,
  and other countries. ASL interpreters on request.
  P.O. Box 85596, Seattle, WA 98105
  (206) 568-7777
  (206) 517-9670 TTY MSG
  Fax (206) 325-2601
  www.aabl.org
  info@aabl.org

Alcoholics Anonymous
  The original 12-step program that has helped
  millions of alcoholics.
  P.O. Box 459, Grand Central Station,
  New York, NY 10163
  (212) 647-1680
  www.alcoholics-anonymous.org

Al-Anon Family Groups
  Support groups for family members of alcoholics.
  P.O. Box 862, Midtown Station,
  New York, NY 10018
  (800) 356-9996
  www.al-anon.org

Boston Women's Health Book Collective
  Authors of *Our Bodies, Ourselves for the New
  Century*. Numerous women's health links.
  www.ourbodiesourselves.org

Callen-Lorde
  Serves the lesbian, gay, bisexual, and transgender
  communities and people living with HIV/AIDS.
  356 West 18th St., New York, NY 10011
  (212) 271-7200
  Fax (212) 271-8111
  www.callen-lorde.org

Center for Sexual Abuse Treatment National Drug
Abuse Hotline
  Information line with referrals to treatment
  programs.
  (800) 662-HELP

The Clitoris.com
  Fascinating site with all sorts of information
  about female sexuality. Links to sources of
  information on anatomy, cancer, disability,
  childbirth, clit pumping, and masturbation.
  www.the-clitoris.com
  webmaster@the-clitoris.com

Co-Dependents Anonymous
  P.O. Box 33577, Phoenix, AZ 85067
  www.codependents.org/index.html
  info@codependents.org

Fenway Community Health Center
  Comprehensive, community-based health care
  clinic.
  7 Haviland St., Boston, MA 02115
  (617) 267-0900
  www.fchc.org

The Healing Woman Foundation
  Dedicated to providing recovery resources for
  women survivors of childhood sexual abuse. "Our
  goal is to create a strong, organized, vocal
  community of women survivors of childhood
  sexual abuse and their supporters who can speak
  out about violence against women and children."
  Publishes *The Healing Woman*, a bimonthly
  newsletter. Sponsors workshops and conferences.
  P.O. Box 28040-C, San Jose, CA 95159
  Tel. (800) 477-4111
  Fax (408) 247-4309
  www.healingwoman.org
  HealingW@healingwoman.org

Kink Aware Professionals
  International referrals to psychotherapeutic,
  medical, dental, complementary healing, and
  legal professionals who are knowledgeable about
  and sensitive to diverse expressions of sexuality.
  All listed professionals have volunteered to be
  available for referral to people involved in "kinky"
  sexuality (leather, S/M, fetish, and the like).
  www.bannon.com/kap

Lesbian Health Information Network (LHINetwork)
A worldwide network for distributing information relating to lesbian health research, education, and services. Serves as a resource and networking tool for those involved in lesbian health.
To subscribe, send a request to
LHINetwork@worldnet.att.net
including your full name, e-mail address, how you heard about the list, and a brief description of your work in lesbian health.
For more information, contact:
Connie Winkle
c/o Health Resource Network of Texas
P.O. Box 150791, Arlington, TX 76015
LHINetwork@worldnet.att.net

Lesbian Health Web Ring
A network of personal web pages dedicated to the health of lesbians and all other women who have sex with women.
www.geocities.com/HotSprings/Spa/2466/webring.html
hope@4wmn.com

LesbianSTD.com
Health information from the Lesbian-Bisexual Women's Health Study at the University of Washington.
www.lesbianstd.com

Lyon-Martin Women's Health Services
Provides comprehensive health care for women by women with a focus on lesbians, women of color, low-income women, older women, and women with disabilities. Conducts forums, workshops, and support groups for lesbian, gay, and bisexual parents and prospective parents.
1748 Market St., Ste. 201,
San Francisco, CA 94102
(415) 565-7667

Mautner Project for Lesbians with Cancer
Direct services to lesbians with cancer, their partners and caregivers as well as community education and advocacy.
1707 L St., NW, Ste. 500
Washington, DC 20036
(202) 332 5536 (Voice/TTY)
Fax (202) 332-0662
www.mautnerproject.org

Narcotics Anonymous
Twelve-step program for people in recovery from drug addiction.
World Service Office, Inc.
P.O. Box 9999, Van Nuys, CA 91409
Tel. (818) 780-3951
Fax (818) 785-0923
www.na.org

Overeaters Anonymous
Twelve-step program for people in recovery from compulsive overeating.
World Service Office
6075 Zenith Ct. N.E., Rio Rancho, NM 87124
Tel. (505) 891-2664
Fax (505) 891-4320
www.overeatersanonymous.org

Sex and Love Addicts Anonymous
Twelve-step program for people in recovery from sex and love addiction.
The Augustine Fellowship
P.O. Box 338, Norwood, MA 02062
(781) 255-8825
www.slaafws.org
slaafws@aol.com

Retail and Mail Order

Many sex-toy stores offer workshops and other programs of interest to lesbian and bisexual women. They also post information about local events. Most retail outlets also welcome mail-order business.

MAIL ORDER ONLY

Adam and Eve
Mail-order catalog of toys, videos, DVDs, books, safer-sex supplies, and lingerie. Web site links to the Sinclair Intimacy Institute, an extensive sex education resource: www.intimacyinstitute.com
P.O. Box 200, Carrboro, NC 27510
(800) 274-0333
(919) 644-1212
www.adameve.com
custserv@adameve.com

Aslan Leather
A woman-owned manufacturer of leather, rubber, and vinyl gear. Dildo harnesses, bondage gear, and whips can be purchased at many of the stores listed here or direct from the manufacturer. The web site picture gallery is well worth the trip!
Box 102, Stn. B, Toronto,
ON M5T 2T3, Canada
(416) 306.0462
www.AslanLeather.com
aslan@interlog.com

Blowfish
Blowfish calls itself "the hippest sex stuff company" on the internet. "Blowfish doesn't just throw whatever products our vendors want us to carry on our web pages. We read the books, watch the videos, play with the toys, squirt the lube; everything we carry is something that we like." Mail-order catalog of toys, books, DVDs, comics, magazines, videos, and safer-sex supplies. Don't miss the What's Cool page.
P.O. Box 411290, San Francisco CA 94141
Tel. (800) 325-2569, (415) 252-4340
Fax (415) 252-4349
www.blowfish.com
blowfish@blowfish.com

Blue Door
Adult video rentals; features a selection of lesbian videos, from *Suburban Dykes* to *Leather Bound Dykes from Hell.*
ETP, Inc.
P.O. Box 64378, Sunnyvale, CA 94089
Fax (408) 733-2372
www.bluedoor.com
blueinfo@bluedoor.com

CDS Bookstand
Books and videos for the transgender community.
www.cdspub.com
JoAnn@cdspub.com

Cetra Latex-Free Supplies
Main order source of nitrile, vinyl, polyurethane safer-sex supplies. Stocks dental dams made from silicone.
888-LATEX NO
(510) 848 3345
www.latexfree.com

The Frugal Domme
Reasonably priced S/M toys. Catalog available for $5.
TFD Enterprises
P.O. Box 581173, Modesto, CA 95358
www.frugaldomme.com
domina@frugaldomme.com

Glyde Dams
Source for safer-sex supplies.
www.sheerglydedams.com

Heartwood Whips of Passion
Janette Heartwood has been making fine floggers, cats, and other whips since 1990. Deerskin, cowhide, elk, horsehair, bullhide, bison, and rubber.
P.O. Box 490, Herndon, VA 20172
(703) 834 0757
www.heartwoodwhips.com
Janette@ heartwoodwhips.com

JT's Stockroom

Carries an impressive line of S/M and bondage gear. Web site features a sizzling gallery with photos of toys and gear modeled by JT's staff.
2140 Hyperion Ave., Los Angeles, CA 90027
Tel. (800) 755-TOYS, (323) 666-2121
Fax (800) 357-8697, (323) 913-5976
www.stockroom.com
info@stockroom.com

Lashes by Sarah

High-quality, hand-crafted cats and floggers in deerskin, cowhide, bullhide, buffalo—from the sensuous to the severe.
P.O. Box 5245, Oakland, CA 94605
(510) 638-3564
www.lashesbysarah.com
lashes@sirius.com

Stompers Boots

Engineer boots, biker boots, lace-up boots, riding boots.
323 10th St., San Francisco, CA 94103
Tel. (415) 255-6422
Fax (415) 863-0456
www.stompersboots.com
info@stompersboots.com

Vixen Creations

Fine art and eroticism meet at Vixen Creations, the women-owned and -operated manufacturer of hand-made silicone dildos and plugs. Visit the web site to order online or to find a Vixen retailer near you.
1004 Revere, Ste. B-49,
San Francisco, CA 94124
Tel. and Fax (415) 822-0403
www.vixencreations.com
VixenSi@sirius.com

Xandria Collection

For 25 years, the Xandria catalog has offered a wide array of vibrators, dildos, lingerie, leather, videos, books, and more. Betty Dodson is on the Xandria advisory board.
165 Valley Dr., Brisbane, CA 94005
(800) 242-2823
(415) 468-3812
www.xandria.com
info@xandria.com

RETAIL STORES

▼ United States

A Woman's Touch

A feminist store operated by Ellen Barnard, M.S.S.W., and Myrtle Wilhite, M.D., M.S., A Woman's Touch offers toys, books, and safer-sex supplies. "We celebrate sexuality and pleasure for women and those who love them." The web site features Ask Aphrodite and Ask Dr. Myrtle with some of the best advice columns you'll find on the Web.
600 Williamson St., Madison, WI 53703
(608) 250-1928
www.a-womans-touch.com
wmstouch@midplains.net

Come Again Erotic Emporium

Woman-owned store offering toys, books, and lingerie, plus book and fetish magazine catalog.
353 E. 53rd St., New York, NY 10022
(212) 308-9394

Condomania

Retail stores and mail-order catalog of condoms and safer-sex supplies. Stocks an extensive array of products, including nonlatex barriers.
7306 Melrose Ave., Los Angeles, CA 90046
(323) 933-7865
351 Bleecker St., New York, NY 10014
(212) 691-9442
www.condomania.com
info@condomania.com

Eve's Garden

Woman-oriented store and catalog of toys, books, and videos.
119 W. 57th St., Ste. #420, New York, NY 10019
(800) 848-3837
(212) 757-8651
www.evesgarden.com
huntress@evesgarden.com

Forbidden Fruit

Every day is Valentine's Day at Forbidden Fruit, a woman-owned and -operated business whose mission is to "help create erotic self-awareness and improve intimate communication in relationships." Operates a toy store, fetish wear boutique, and body modification studio.

Toy Store and Educational Center
512 Neches St., Austin, TX 78701
(512) 478-8358

Fetish Boutique
108 E. North Loop Blvd., Austin, TX 78751
(512) 453-8090

Body Art Salon
513 E. Sixth St., Austin, TX 78701
(512) 476-4596
www.forbiddenfruit.com
info@forbiddenfruit.com

Good Vibrations

Promoting sexual pleasure since 1977. "At Good Vibrations, we believe that sexual pleasure is everyone's birthright, and that access to sexual materials and accurate sex information promotes health and happiness. Our goal is to serve as a resource for quality products and information, to model honest communication about sexuality, and to take every possible opportunity to promote the philosophy that sex is fun and natural. We hope you'll join us in our pursuit of pleasure!" Two retail locations and a mail-order catalog of books, toys, and videos. Check the web site for the after-hours schedule of store events.

Stores:
1210 Valencia St., San Francisco, CA 94110
(415) 974-8980
2504 San Pablo Ave., Berkeley, CA 94702
(510) 841-8987

Mail-order:
938 Howard St., Ste. 101,
San Francisco, CA 94103
(800) 289-8423
(415) 974-8990
www.goodvibes.com
goodvibe@well.com

Grand Opening!

"No matter what your persuasion, you're always welcome at Grand Opening! Since we've been open, thousands of people have visited and have been made to feel at home in our cozy little boutique. We are hoping you'll enjoy the same homey atmosphere when visiting us from your desktop or laptop!" Offers many workshops and other events. Retail store and mail-order catalog of books, toys, and videos.

318 Harvard St., Ste. 32, Arcade Bldg.,
Coolidge Corner, Brookline, MA 02446
Toll-free ordering line: (877) 731-2626
Tel. (617) 731-2626
Fax (617) 731-2693
www.grandopening.com
grando@grandopening.com

Passionflower

Erotica store.
4 Yosemite Ave., Oakland, CA 94611
(510) 601-7750

Pleasure Chest

Retail store and catalog of toys and clothing.
7733 Santa Monica Blvd.,
West Hollywood, CA 90046
(800) 75-DILDO, mail-order
(213) 650-1022, store
www.thepleasurechest.com

Purple Passion

Toys, magazines, books, boots, corsets, and other fetish clothing for men and women—rubber, leather, chain mail, patent leather, and PVC. Latex clothing by Naughty Nancy, toys by Jean and Kate, and chain mail from Sonya Blaze. A full line of BDSM and sex toys. Stocks, whips, and toys from Janette Heartwood, Lashes by Sarah, Sorodz, Elizabeth Gonzalez, and other women toymakers. "We have rated most of our impact toys, ranging from 1, which is soft and sensuous, to 5, which is heavy and severe." Yeow!
242 W. 16th St., New York, NY 10011
Tel. (212) 807-0486
Fax (212) 807-7582
www.purplepassion.com
ppassion1@aol.com
info@purplepassion.com

Rubber Tree
  Retail store for safer-sex supplies.
  4426 Burke Avenue No., Seattle, WA 98103
  (206) 663-4750

Spartacus Leathers
  300 S.W. 12th Ave., Portland, OR 97205
  (503) 224-2604

Stormy Leather
  "A San Francisco landmark for 15 years, Stormy
  Leather is a woman-owned company dedicated
  to providing the highest quality garments and
  toys. There is something for everyone here:
  beginners, intermediate players, and pros."
  Specializes in leather and PVC fetish wear. Known
  for its beautiful corsets and attractive, durable
  dildo harnesses. Hosts events in its San Francisco
  store.
  1158 Howard St., San Francisco, CA 94103
  (415) 626-1672
  www.stormyleather.com

Toys in Babeland
  A sex-toy shop run by women, dedicated to
  providing women and others the support,
  information, and equipment they want to have
  fun and fulfilling sex lives. "We sell sex toys to
  make money, make friends, and change the
  world. We share a belief in every person's right
  to define their own sexuality and gender, and to
  pursue pleasure in any way that does not harm
  others. We are S/M, transgender, queer, straight,
  vanilla, and bi friendly." Retail stores and catalog
  of toys, books, and videos.
  (800) 658-9119
  www.babeland.com
  biglove@babeland.com
  Stores:
    711 E. Pike St., Seattle, WA 98122
    (206) 328-2914
    94 Rivington St., New York, NY 10002
    (212) 375-1701

▼ Canada

Come As You Are
  Cooperatively owned store and mail-order catalog
  of toys, books, and videos. Web site features resources
  on sex and disability. "Our approach to sexuality
  is one of respect, openness, humor, communication,
  and responsibility. We are service- and community-
  oriented. We are accessible and disability-positive.
  Nous offrons des services limités en français."
  701 Queen St. W., Toronto, ON, M6J 1E6, Canada
  Toll-free: (877) 858-3160
  (416) 504-7934
  www.comeasyouare.com
  mail@comeasyouare.com

Good for Her
  "Toronto's cozy, comfortable place where women
  and their admirers can find a variety of high-
  quality sex toys, books, seminars, sensual art, and
  much more." Wheelchair accessible.
  171 Harbord St., Toronto, ON, M5S 1H5, Canada
  Toll-free: (877) 588-0900
  (416) 588-0900
  www.goodforher.com
  whats@goodforher.com

Lovecraft
  Retail stores and online catalog of toys, books,
  videos, and lingerie.
  63 Yorkville Ave.,
  Toronto, ON, M5R 1B7, Canada
  Tel. (416) 923-7331
  Fax (416) 923-4610
  2200 Dundas St.,
  East Mississauga, ON, L4X 2V3, Canada
  (905) 276-5772
  www.lovecraft.inter.net

Womyn's Ware
  Retail store and catalog of toys, books, and fetish
  gear. "Products, services, and an environment for
  the celebration and empowerment of women's
  sexuality." Strong emphasis on education.
  896 Commercial Dr.,
  Vancouver, BC, V5L 3Y5, Canada
  Toll-free (888) WYM-WARE (996-9273)
  Fax (604) 254-5472
  www.womynsware.com
  info@womynsware.com

▼ Europe

SH!
A women's sex shop.
22 Coronet St., London N1, U.K.
Tel. (0171) 613 5458

Tiberius
Leather Latex and Tools
Wien 7, Lindengassw 2, Austria
Tel. 43 1 522 04 74
www.tiberius.at
leather@tiberius.at

Safer-Sex Resources

American Social Health Association
P.O. Box 13827, Research Triangle Park,
NC 27709
(919) 361-8400

Centers for Disease Control National AIDS
Clearinghouse
P.O. Box 6003, Rockville, MD 20849
(800) 342-AIDS
www.cdcnac.com

LesbianSTD.com
www.lesbianstd.com

National AIDS Hotline
(800) 342-2437

National STD Hotline
(800) 227-8922

Planned Parenthood
(800) 230-PLAN
www.ppfa.org

Safer Sex Page:
www.safersex.org

San Francisco Sex Information
Free information and referral switchboard
providing anonymous, accurate, nonjudgmental
information about sex.
(415) 989-SFSI

STD home page:
www.grin.net/~sycamore/std/index.html

BDSM Organizations and Play Parties

The National Leather Association International
NLA-I is an educational group open to kink people
of all genders and sexual orientations. Web site provides links to many S/M organizations and resources.
PMB 155, 3439 N.E. Sandy Blvd.,
Portland, OR 97232
www.nla-i.com

Scene USA
Listing of BDSM organizations in the United
States. Scene USA lists BDSM groups, clubs,
nightclubs, and munches (think: potluck in
fetish gear) by city and state. Lists gay, straight,
and pansexual resources. Cruise for contacts or
submit news of your BDSM community.
www.darkheart.com/sceneusa.html
webmaster@darkheart.com

UNITED STATES

▼ Arizona

Arizona Amazons
For women who have a positive interest in BDSM.
Monthly educational, informational, and social
events in Phoenix. Members must be at least 18.
(602) 669-1000
www.geocities.com/WestHollywood/Heights/323
1/index.html
azamazon@juno.com

▼ California

AWOL
All Women of Leather
Hosts play parties in the San Francisco Bay Area.
Xantasia@aol.com

Castlebar
The Castlebar is a well-equipped dungeon in San
Francisco. Damion Kelley, the Castlebar's
proprietrix, hosts regular play parties. Genetic
and transsexual women may request to join her
e-mail list to receive play party invitations and
announcements.
www.castlebar.com
damion@best.com

The Exiles
A social and educational organization in San Francisco for women with a positive personal interest in S/M between women. Publishes a monthly newsletter. Monthly educational and social events, details of local play parties.
P.O. Box 31266, San Francisco, CA 94131
(415) 487-5170
www.theexiles.org
exiles@theexiles.org

House of Differences
A different kind of B&B—bed & bondage (Elizabeth doesn't do breakfast). Five bedrooms plus Elizabeth's safe, elegant San Francisco dungeon. Differences hosts regular play parties, as well as educational seminars and workshops.
www.differences.com
Elizabeth@differences.com

LA RAWW
Los Angeles Radical And Wicked Women is an educational and social group serving Los Angeles, Orange, Riverside, and San Bernardino counties. The group meets monthly on the fourth Saturday at a local dungeon in the Silverlake area of L.A. Demonstrations or discussions are followed by play in the dungeon. Topics for meetings range widely. The group is open to women, men with feminine persona, and transgendered people ages 18 and over. A $5 donation is requested for the meeting and an additional $5 for the play party.
(800) 866-3983
LARAWW@aol.com

L.A.S.H.
The Leather and Sisterhood Club for leatherwomen in Southern California, a women's BDSM club that meets monthly. L.A.S.H. is open to the women of Southern California, and is supportive of all women—lesbians, women in transition, and transgendered, heterosexual, and bisexual women.
(619) 364-5274
l_a_s_h@yahoo.com
homepages.go.com/~l_a_s_h

Queen of Heaven
Carol Queen's infamous San Francisco play parties are open to invited guests and their guests. "QOH is a pansexual pagan event, although an attendee need not identify as either pansexual or pagan; s/he simply must be comfortable enough sharing an erotic space with others." Safe-sex rules apply. To get on the party list, contact Queen at: 2215-R Market St., Ste. 455, San Francisco CA 94114 or CarolQueen@aol.com

▼ Florida

SLLAP (Southern Leather Lesbians At Play)
SLLAP offers social events, educational demos, lectures, and an opportunity to meet, play with, and network with other leather lesbians. Meetings are open to any female over 21, regardless of sexual preference. Membership open to lesbians over 21 years old.
P.O. Box 24753, Ft. Lauderdale, FL 33307
(954) 463-6251
www.gate.net/~ldlmaam/sllap.htm
SLLAP@aol.com

▼ Georgia

Southern Women's Power Exchange
Hosts play parties in Atlanta.
Contact: DaddiDuir@aol.com (type "SWPE" in the subject line of your e-mail)

▼ Iowa, Missouri, Nebraska

Janet R. is the contact person for "an informal kinky co-op of women" in Kansas City, Des Moines, Omaha, and Lincoln who host play parties for women and trans people. "We have successfully included trans people, FTM as well as MTF, even pre-op (you have to love small communities for that!)." Contact Janet R. at:
P.O. Box 32732, Kansas City, MO 64171
(816) 523-4154
photojan@aol.com

▼ Maryland

FIST

Females Investigating Sexual Terrain

Open to women 21 years of age or older who are interested in S/M, leather, or fetish sex between women. FIST has a snail-mail newsletter and also sends frequent e-mail notices about upcoming events of interest to women. FIST does not host parties, but does help publicize parties for women that take place in the Mid-Atlantic area.

P.O. Box 41032, Baltimore, MD 21203

(410) 385-8686

members.aol.com/FISTWomen

FISTWomen@aol.com

Play House Studios and Gallery

An erotic art gallery, fetish photography studio, and award-winning play space in Baltimore, Md. Open to any person over the age of 21. Play House produces a monthly snail-mail calendar of events, sends e-mail reminders about upcoming events, and uses its web page to disseminate information. "Most of our parties are pansexual and women are most welcome! We also host quarterly women-only parties and over the Thanksgiving weekend we host Just Play—a weekend of play for women."

P.O. Box 22185. Baltimore, MD 21203

Tel. (410) 332-1802

Fax (410) 332-1848

www.kitco.net/playhouse

PlayHse@aol.com

▼ Massachusetts

MOB (Massachusetts Orgasmic Bitches)

The MOB is an exciting, sexy, fun, and diverse group of women who are interested in S/M between women. MOB welcomes all women aged 21 and over who want to participate in BDSM—including genetic females (irrespective of gender expression) and MTFs (irrespective of genital surgery). Hosts regular social events. Sign up for the MOB e-mail or snail-mail list.

P.O. Box 790, West Springfield, MA 01090

members.aol.com/boynic/MOB.html

BostonMOB@aol.com

▼ New Mexico

WEST (Women Exploring S/M Themes)

Open to women of all sexual orientations, including transgendered women living full-time as women. Occasionally hosts play parties. Contact Diva Marie, c/o D Major, at:

P.O. Box 36287, Albuquerque, NM 87176

(505) 254-1768

www.divamarie.com/group.htm

divamarie@mindspring.com

▼ New York

Bound and Determined (B.A.D. Women)

BDSM support group for women in the Albany, New York, area. Available to any women over 18 years old of any sexual orientation.

(518) 221-3922

www.fetishnetwork.com/BAD

blindspt@capital.net

Dyke Uniform Corps (DUC)

A private association of women of honor, integrity, and discipline ("Yes, ma'am!") whose mission is to explore common interests in wearing military and law enforcement uniforms within the S/M, leather, and fetish communities.

DUCNY@aol.com

members.aol.com/ducny

Fireball Productions

Hosts leatherdyke play parties in New York City.

(718) 788-5122

fireballmc@aol.com

Lesbian Sex Mafia

Founded in 1981, LSM is a support and information group for lesbian, bisexual, heterosexual, and transsexual women interested in S/M. Sign up for e-mail announcements:

www.onelist.com/subscribe.cgi/lsm-nyc

members.aol.com/lpnnyc/lsm.html

lsmnyc@hotmail.com

TES Women's Group

The Eulenspiegel Society of New York is one of the oldest S/M groups in North America. The TES Women's Group's purpose is to network, socialize, and share knowledge and experiences among sisters in the BDSM scene.
www.tes.org/welcome.html
tes@tes.org

▼ Ohio

Briar Rose

The Briar Rose group offers activities and associations in Columbus.
janhall@hotmail.com

▼ Oregon

Leatherwomen's Supper Club is a group of women in Portland who are interested in or participate in S/M activities and who get together once a month for a potluck dinner. No dues, no orientation meetings, no workshops, no play parties, no by-laws, and no politics—just women who share a common interest in getting together to socialize and share a meal.
lynnes@teleport.com

Lulu's Pervy Playhouse

A group for S/M women from Portland and the surrounding area. Open to women 18 years of age or older, lesbians, bisexuals, heterosexuals, and transgender women who identify as female. Hosts monthly play parties.
www.jps.net/wynter/luluspage.html
lululist@hotmail.com
wynter@bigfoot.com

▼ Pennsylvania

Labrys Play Group

Hosts women-only play parties in a fully equipped dungeon space in Philadelphia. Contact Marya at:
maryasub@aol.com

Pittsburgh LeatherGrrrls

Open to all women (those having XX chromosomes or living as women 24/7) who are interested in kinky play and discussions on S/M safety, edge play, role-playing, emotional aspects of kink, and transgender issues. LeatherGrrrls hosts an e-mail list for news and discussions. Welcomes contact with women traveling through the Pittsburgh area and who live nearby. Many of the LeatherGrrrls participate in the Pittsburgh Munch group, a pansexual organization that hosts dinners and workshops. Contact c/o Gay and Lesbian Community Center
(412) 422-0114
LeatherGrrrls-request@charcoal.com

▼ Texas

Bound by Desire

For lesbian, bisexual, heterosexual, and transsexual women interested in dominance and submission and S/M. Monthly educational, informational, and social events in Austin.
P.O. Box 3733, Austin, TX 78704
www.merrymeet.com/bbd
BoundbyDesire91@juno.com

Dyke Uniform Corps (DUC)

A private association of women of honor, integrity, and discipline ("Yes, Ma'am!") whose mission is to explore common interests in wearing military and law enforcement uniforms within the S/M, leather, and fetish communities.
P.O. Box 691025, San Antonio, TX 78269
members.aol.com/ducny
DUC NY@aol.com

▼ Virginia

The Black Rose

A pansexual support, education, and social group for adults who share an interest in expressions of power in love and play, including D/S (dominance and submission), B/D (bondage and discipline), fetishism, and cross-dressing. You must be over 21 to attend functions.
P.O. Box 11161, Arlington, VA 22210
www.br.org
br@br.org

▼ Washington

Sisters of Sin
  Seattle-based social group for women interested
  in participating in BDSM. Hosts workshops and
  other events. Open to women 18 and over with
  female ID.
  www.byz.org/~sos/index.html
  sos@byz.org

The Wet Spot: Seattle's Sex Positive
Community Center
  The Wet Spot provides meeting and event space
  for sex-positive organizations. Events include
  regular women-only parties as well as meetings
  and workshops. Details about specific events are
  available on the web site. Membership is
  required for some events. You must be over 18 to
  attend events at The Wet Spot.
  www.wetspot.org
  wetspot@bent.org

The Women's Welcoming Committee (WWC)
  A Seattle-based group founded in 1995 to assist
  women over 18 of any sexual orientation who
  are looking for information about BDSM.
  Meetings provide an orientation to local
  resources, information about upcoming events,
  and an opportunity to ask questions. The WWC
  meets the first Tuesday of every month from 7 to
  9 P.M. at The Wet Spot, 1414 W. Garfield.
  www.bent.org/wwc
  johonna@jetcity.com

▼ Wisconsin

Bad Grrrls
  A support group for women who do S/M in
  Madison. Contact A Woman's Touch (see
  "Retail and Mail Order") for current
  information.

Satyricon
  Pansexual, pangender BDSM social group in
  Madison. For more information, contact Ellen
  Barnard at A Woman's Touch (see "Retail and
  Mail Order").

CANADA

Bound
  Sponsors women-only BDSM parties in the
  Vancouver BC area
  Contact: boundbc@hotmail.com

The Women's Bath House Committee
  Hosts Pride Pussy: A Women's Bath House
  Night, an occasional event held at Club Toronto
  in Toronto, Ontario.
  For more information or child-care networking:
  (416) 350-8484, ext. 319
  pussypalace.ets.net
  pussy_palace@hotmail.com

EUROPE

For more information about European resources,
subscribe to Leather Letters, an occasional e-mail
newsletter about woman-to-woman S/M. The
emphasis of Leather Letters is on European events,
but it also contains news from other continents. To
subscribe, contact: tania@xs4all.nl

▼ Austria

Sadomasochismus in Österreich
  Austria's pansexual S/M group; web site features
  links to other European S/M resources.
  www.bdsm.at
  sadonis@bdsm.at

Schlagfertig
  Vienna's monthly women-only BDSM gathering,
  organized by Helene, founder of a women-only
  BDSM mailing list for German-speaking
  members. Web site in German.
  www.datenschlag.org/schlagfertig
  helene@bdsm.at

▼ France

Les Maudites Femelles (LMF)
  c/o Nathalie Dalla Corte
  13 rue Beautreillis, 75004 Paris, France

▼ Germany

Knights of the Round Table
Hosts play parties in Hamburg.
Die_Tafelrunde@hotmail.com

Lifeguard
Support network for S/M women.
www.mela.de/Frauen
neuce@informatik.uni-muenchen.de

SchMacht!
Germany's nationwide network of bisexual and
lesbian women (including transgender people)
interested in BDSM. Publishes newsletter and
hosts play parties and educational events.
stadt.gay-web.de/schmacht
schmacht@gay-web.de

▼ The Netherlands

Wild Side
The only woman-to-woman group in the
Netherlands. Wild Side welcomes women with
extremely varied S/M interests—beginning
players, novices, old-guard leatherdykes, poly
bi-girls, professional sex workers, and straight
women with a taste for playing with women.
Transsexual women are welcome as well. Wild
Side hosts workshops and play parties.

Wild Side News is published five times a year.
A subscription within the Netherlands costs fl
10,- for a year; for the rest of Europe it's fl 15,- by
Eurocheck; for the U.S. it's $10 U.S. personal
check.
Rozenstraat 14, 1016 NX Amsterdam, The
Netherlands
Tel. +31-(0)71-5128632 (Tania)
www.dds.nl\~wildside
Wild Side News subscriptions: arnold@bart.nl
General coordination: tania@xs4all.nl

▼ Sweden

LASH
The club for women who like it rough.
Established in 1995 in Stockholm. Lash
welcomes all women dykes, lesbians, bisexuals,
transsexuals. Publishes 10 newsletters per year;
sends e-mail announcements of events. Hosts
monthly play parties.
c/o SLM Stockholm
Box 172 41, 104 62 Stockholm, Sweden
Tel. 4673-992 62 82
www.welcome.to/clublash
clublash@hotmail.com

▼ United Kingdom

Informed Consent
Web site packed with information on the BDSM
community in the U.K., including events,
personal ads, and a listing of organizations.
P.O. Box 152, Manchester, England M20 2YZ
www.informedconsent.co.uk
webmaster@informedconsent.co.uk

S/M Dykes
A relaxed and very friendly group of woman and
trans men interested in S/M with women. Meets
on the first Tuesday evening of each month at
Central Station Pub, 37 Wharfedale Rd.,
London N1 (Kings Cross tube). For more info
about the British scene contact:
tart@trace1.demon.co.uk

Sex Education Workshops, Classes, and Resources

Body Electric
Committed to helping people experience their potential as healers of self and others through touch, conscious breath, and honoring the wisdom of the body. Offers women-only classes, such as "Celebrating the Body Erotic for Women" and "Sacred Wrestling for Women," in Seattle, Oakland, New York City, and Los Angeles.
6527-A Telegraph Ave., Oakland, CA 94609
Tel. (510) 653-1594
Fax (510) 653-4991
www.bodyelectric.org/women_index.htm
bodyelec@aol.com

The Fairy Butch Dynasty
Karlyn Lotney (aka Fairy Butch) offers ongoing sex ed classes in San Francisco.
www.fairybutch.com
fb@fairybutch.com

San Francisco Sex Information
Offers a 55-hour training course in all aspects of human sexuality, in a positive, supportive atmosphere.
www.sfsi.org

Web Resources

AltSex
Comprehensive site with information on all aspects of BDSM.
www.altsex.org

Bodyart FAQ
www.cis.ohio-state.edu/text/faq/usenet/bodyart/top.html

Dyke Planet
Pour les filles de Dyke PlaNET. Le premier site lesbien français.
www.dykeplanet.com
redac@dykeplanet.com

Dykesworld
Gateway resource for information on lesbian and bisexual women's sexuality, with links to general resources. Offering arts, erotica, interactive areas, personals, cartoons, cyber-postcards by lesbian artists, classifieds and a lot more. All services are free and provided as a work of love and compassion for the lesbian community and its friends.
www.dykesworld.de

FeMiNa
A comprehensive, searchable directory of links to female-friendly sites and information on the World Wide Web.
www.femina.cybergrrl.com
femina@cybergrrl.com

IRC Help
www.irchelp.org

Jane's Net Sex Guide
Jane reviews hundreds of web sites featuring "erotica, sexuality resources, escort services, telephone sex services, fiction, reality, art, anime, and alternative lifestyles."
www.janesguide.com/index.html

QueerNet
Provides dozens of e-mail discussion lists for the gay, lesbian, bisexual, transgendered, and S/M communities (see below). The web site gives detailed information on how to subscribe to the lists, which include many supportive lists for women exploring all facets of sexuality and gender. (You can start your own list, too, with the enthusiastic support of the folks at QueerNet.org!)
www.queernet.org

SIECUS (Sexuality Information and Education Council of the United States)
SIECUS develops, collects, and disseminates information on sexuality, promotes comprehensive education about sexuality, and advocates the right of individuals to make responsible sexual choices.
130 W. 42nd St., Ste. 350, New York, NY 10036
Tel. (212) 819-9770
Fax (212) 819-9776
siecus@siecus.org

Society for Human Sexuality

A comprehensive online library of sexuality
resources—one of the most useful sites on the
Web. The Society for Human Sexuality is a
social and educational organization devoted to
the appreciation of the myriad consensual forms
of human relationships and sexual expression.
Offers lectures and other programs in Seattle.
PMB 1276, 1122 E. Pike St., Seattle, WA 98122
www.sexuality.org
shs@sexuality.org

Web by Women for Women

A group of sex-positive, anticensorship feminists
created this site to give voice to women's stories
about sex, contraception, menstruation,
pregnancy, and sexual identity.
www.io.com/~wwwomen/sexuality/index.html

The Womb

Perhaps the most beautiful lesbian site on the
Web.
womb.wwdc.com/tunnels.html

MAILING LISTS

You can find an e-mail discussion list to match just
about any interest you can imagine. Many of the lists
below are hosted by QueerNet, which provides a
wonderful service by supporting mailing lists for the
gay, lesbian, bisexual, transgendered, and BDSM communities. The 200 QueerNet lists serve more than
36,000 subscribers. QueerNet is supported entirely
by donations. The complete list of lists (with tech-
nical instructions) can be found at: www.queernet.org.
Queer.org.au Inc., an Australian queer community
resource, also maintains lists of interest to lesbians
and bisexual women (some of which you'll find
below). The complete roster of Queer.org.au lists
(for queers of all genders) can be found at:
lists.queer.org.au or admin@queer.org.au

Lesbian.org maintains the mother of all lesbian lists!
www.lesbian.org/lesbian-lists
sappho@sappho.net

Joan Korenman maintains a list of "gender-related"
lists.
www.umbc.edu/wmst/forums.html
korenman@umbc2.umbc.edu

Amazon Alternatives in Healing

A self-help support e-mail group for lesbian
survivors of childhood sexual abuse. AAIH
provides "a safe, supportive environment within
which group members can share their feelings
and experiences with each other, in a
nonjudgmental and understanding way."
For information, contact:
owner-aaih@queernet.org
To subscribe, send an e-mail to
majordomo@queernet.org
In the body of the e-mail, type:
subscribe aaih <your e-mail address>

American Boyz

American Boyz hosts a number of mailing lists:
Amboyz-Main (general e-mail list), Amboyz-
Latino (Latino issues), Amboyz-Faith
(discussions of spirituality), Alamo Boyz (Texas),
Dezertboyz (Tucson and southern Arizona),
Metro-DC (Virginia; Washington, D.C.;
Maryland), Midwest Boyz (Midwest), SOFFA-ACT
(significant others, friends, families, and allies),
ElderTG (over 50). Info and help about mailing
lists can be obtained by sending e-mail to:
listwrangler@iximd.com or
amboyz@iximd.com

Badgirls

A discussion list for women who do S/M with
other women. The list is designed to be a social
and educational forum about BDSM, leather,
fetishes, and role play. Membership is limited to
adult women (bisexual, straight/heterosexual,
lesbian, queer, transgendered, transsexual) who
have a positive interest in this type of play with
women. "In addition to networking and sharing
information, we hope to facilitate personal
relationships between leatherwomen... and to
get girls dates!" The list is closed and private. It
is also a list with a strong focus on Australia and
New Zealand, but has subscribers from all over
the world.
For more information or to subscribe:
lists.queer.org.au/mailman/listinfo.cgi/badgirls

Black-LatinoNYCNJ

For gay and lesbian blacks and Latinos in the
greater New York City/New Jersey area. Have a
chat, find a date or a mate, or just have some fun.
For information, contact:
bkljcnj1@yahoo.com

Boychicks

For butches, femmes, and their supporters.
Boychicks is about butch identity, femme identity,
relationships, and gender issues. Boychicks is
S/M and kink-friendly and sex-positive.
For information, contact:
   boychicks-owner@queernet.org
To subscribe, send an e-mail to
   majordomo@queernet.org
In the body of the e-mail, type:
   subscribe boychicks <your e-mail address>

Butch-Femme

A list where femmes and butches may talk freely
with each other about butch–femme
relationships and issues in a butch–femme
environment.
For information, contact:
   owner-butch-femme @queernet.org
To subscribe, send an e-mail to
   majordomo@queernet.org
In the body of the e-mail, type:
   subscribe butch-femme <your e-mail address>

CFS-GLB

Chronic Fatigue Syndrome G/L/B
For the discussion of issues facing gays, lesbians,
and bisexuals who are afflicted with Chronic
Fatigue Syndrome, fibromyalgia, Multiple Chemical
Sensitivities, or Gulf War Syndrome. CFS-GLB
provides a supportive atmosphere to "share
experiences, vent frustrations and fears, ask
questions, lend and receive help from each other,
and hopefully form friendships in the process."
For information, contact:
   owner-cfs-glb @queernet.org
To subscribe, send an e-mail to
   majordomo@queernet.org
In the body of the e-mail, type:
   subscribe cfs-glb <your e-mail address>

Cyber-Butch-Femme

A list for butches and femmes who identify as lesbians, women, and/or females to freely talk with
each other in a friendly and respectful atmosphere. All butch–femme topics will be allowed.
For information, contact:
   owner-cyber-butch-femme@queer.org.au
To subscribe, send an e-mail to
   majordomo@queer.org.au
In the body of the e-mail, type:
   subscribe cyber-butch-femme <your e-mail
   address>

Deaf Queer Digest

For information, contact:
   owner-deaf-queer-digest@queernet.org
To subscribe, send an e-mail to
   majordomo@queernet.org
In the body of the e-mail, type:
   subscribe deaf-queer-digest <your e-mail
   address>

Disabled-Bi

For disabled bisexuals who want to chat "in an
atmosphere of understanding and love. Disabled, in
regards to this list, means any physical or emotional
ailment that impairs your standard of life. We
welcome anyone who is disabled or any bisexual
that has to live or deal with a disabled person."
For information, contact:
   owner- disabled-bi @queernet.org
To subscribe, send an e-mail to
   majordomo@queernet.org
In the body of the e-mail, type:
   subscribe disabled-bi <your e-mail address>

DisAbledPervs

For discussion of issues related to BDSM and disabilities. It is for people with disabilities who are
interested in BDSM, as well as play partners and
others who would like to help make the leather/
BDSM community more accessible to people with
disabilities. You can subscribe to the list on the
onelist.com web site; however, the list owner requests that you simultaneously send her an e-mail
introducing yourself. Please describe your interest
in disAbledPervs and tell how you heard of the list.
For information, contact list owner:
   disAbledpevs-owner@onelist.com
To subscribe:
   www.onelist.com

Dyke Planet

   Les filles de Dyke PlaNET. Le premier site lesbien français.

   www.dykeplanet.com/

   redac@dykeplanet.com

Euro-Sappho

   For Sapphic discussion on topics of interest to
European dykes. While any woman can join, sub-
scribers should keep in mind the international/
European nature of the list. Current subscribers
reside in Australia, Austria, Belgium, Brazil, Canada,
Denmark, Egypt, Estonia, Finland, France, Germany,
Greece, Hungary, Ireland, Israel, Italy, Luxembourg,
the Netherlands, New Zealand, Norway, Poland,
Portugal, Serbia, Spain, Sweden, Switzerland,
Turkey, U.K., and U.S. The list information is
available in English, French, German, and Spanish.

   For information, contact:

      euro-sappho-request@sappho.net

   www.sappho.net/euro-sappho

FatGrrl Sex

   A social and educational forum about general
sexual expression, BDSM, leather, fetishes, and
role-play for women who are fat-positive, queer,
prosex, and prokink. Membership is limited to
adult women/females (bisexual, straight/
heterosexual, lesbian, butch, femme, queer,
transgendered, transsexual) who have a positive
interest in this type of sexual expression with
other women.

   For information, contact:

      miranda@interlog.com or

      webmaster@queercanada.com

   www.interlog.com/~miranda/fgs

Femmedykes

   For fem(me)s who partner with butches, TGs,
TSs, and FTMs. Femme lesbians/bi-dykes and
butch friends and admirers are welcome to join.

   For information, contact:

      femmedykes-owner @queernet.org

   To subscribe, send an e-mail to

      majordomo@queernet.org

   In the body of the e-mail, type:

      subscribe femmedykes <your e-mail address>

GL-ASB

   Gay/Lesbian Alt.Sex.Bondage

   For discussion of B/D, D/S, and S/M interests
and practices involving same-sex partners.

   For information, contact:

      owner-gl-asb@queernet.org

   To subscribe, send an e-mail to

      majordomo@queernet.org

   In the body of the e-mail, type:

      subscribe gl-asb <your e-mail address>

Kinky-Girls

   For women who do S/M with other women. A
social and educational forum about BDSM,
leather, fetishes, and role-play. Membership is
limited to adult women (bisexual, straight/
heterosexual, lesbian, queer, transgendered,
transsexual) who have a positive interest in this
type of play with other women. This list is
private and new subscribers generally must be
referred by a current list member. If you do not
know anyone on the list you can write to the list
owners <kinky-girls-owner@queernet.org>and
make a personal application. You must provide
your full legal name, age, gender, location, and
information about your interests/experience in
BDSM. In some cases telephone verification will
be required.

   For information, contact:

      kinky-girls-owner@queernet.org

   To subscribe, send an e-mail to

      majordomo@queernet.org

   In the body of the e-mail, type:

      subscribe kinky-girls firstname lastname <your
e-mail address>

Lesbian Cancer List

For lesbian and bisexual women (regardless of birth gender) who wish to discuss the impact of cancer in their lives—women who have or who have had cancer, as well as partners, family, and friends of people with cancer. Health care practitioners working in this field are also welcome.

For information, contact:
    owner-lcl@queernet.org   or
    falcngrl@durham.net   or
    shadowlf@durham.net
To subscribe, send an e-mail to
    majordomo@queernet.org
In the body of the e-mail, type:
    subscribe lcl <your e-mail address>

Living

For lesbian and bisexual women with disabilities, and women who love them, whether lovers, friends, sisters, moms, or daughters.
Although discussion of sex is not discouraged, it is not the primary focus of the list.
For information, send an e-mail to
    majordomo@queernet.org
In the body of the e-mail, type: info living

Long-Distance Dykes

For dykes who are in long-distance relationships. Fairly central are issues of immigration, relocating, monogamy vs. nonmonogamy, killing time without killing the relationship, making transitions to living together full time (or to being apart), and "Are we crazy to be doing this?"
For information, contact:
    long-distance-dykes -owner@queernet.org
To subscribe, send an e-mail to
    majordomo@queernet.org
In the body of the e-mail, type:
    subscribe long-distance-dykes <your e-mail address>

Nice Jewish Girls

A wide-ranging, unmoderated, and tolerant discussion of issues of interest to Jewish lesbian and bisexual women.
For information, contact the list owners:
    lhava@mcs.net
To subscribe, send an e-mail to
    listproc@shamash.org
In the body of the e-mail, type:
    subscribe nicejg firstname lastname <your e-mail address>

OAmazons

For lesbians seeking and sharing experience, ideas, and solutions in regard to eating disorders.
For information, contact the
    OAmazons-owner@queernet.org
To subscribe, send an e-mail to
    majordomo@queernet.org
In the body of the e-mail, type:
    subscribe oamazons firstname lastname <your e-mail address>

OWLS (Older Wiser Lesbians)

For lesbians 40 and older, a place for conversation, friendship, and support. OWLs strives to maintain a space that will feel safe to all, including women who are new to lesbian life and/or new to e-mail discussion lists.
For information, send an e-mail to:
    majordomo@queernet.org
In the body of the e-mail, type: info owls

Poly-Dykes

A women-only list for discussion of the "problems, joys, and general issues that arise in the practice of nonexclusive relationships between women." Welcomes both lesbians and bisexual women. "Poly refers to the practice of being open to having sexual/romantic relationships with more than one woman at a time, and includes relationships models like polyamory, polyfidelity, nonmonogamy, and open relationships."
For information, send e-mail to
    majordomo@queernet.org
In the body of the e-mail, type: info poly-dykes

Queergirlies

For young women (ages 15 to 25) with disabilities who are lesbian, bisexual, or transgendered, from any background, race, or religion. "We discuss issues that we deal with on a daily basis, such as coming out, sex, etc."
For information, contact:
owner-queergirlies@gimpgirl.com   or
lists@gimpgirl.com

Sexpanic

For discussion of the harassment and closure of sex clubs, bathhouses, and public sex spaces; racist selective enforcement and policing of lesbian/gay bars; antisex AIDS activism and education campaigns; increased policing of and attacks on sex workers; and the burgeoning demonizing of sex in current gay men's writings.
For information, contact:
owner-sexpanic@queernet.org
To subscribe, send an e-mail to
majordomo@queernet.org
In the body of the e-mail, type:
subscribe sexpanic <your e-mail address>

Sistahnet!

For lesbian, bisexual, bi-curious, and transgendered women of African descent aged 18 and older. "It is a place to learn, expand, share experiences, and explore a full range of emotions from tears to laughter. Whether you sit on the porch and listen awhile or just want to talk— wipe your feet off and pull up a chair!"
For information, contact:
sistanet@queernet.org   or
demeter.hampshire.edu/~sistah/

Soberdykes

Offers support for lesbian and bisexual women in recovery from alcohol or drug dependence. "You can talk about anything here, from working your program to programs that don't work; taking it one day at a time to celebrating years of sobriety."
For information, contact:
soberdykes-owner@queernet.org
To subscribe, send an e-mail to
majordomo@queernet.org
In the body of the e-mail, type:
subscribe soberdykes firstname lastname <your e-mail address>

Stonebutch

For butches and their femme admirers. The list is for discussion of butch and stone butch issues and butch/femme relationships.
For information, contact:
daddyrhon@earthlink.net
www.butch-femme.com/stonebutch
To subscribe, go to:
lists.queer.org.au/mailman/listinfo.cgi/stonebutch

Stonefemme

A close-knit community of female-born femmes who are partnered or desire to be partnered with butches. Support, community, and a safe place in which to discuss issues of interest to femmes… "and more specifically femme issues as they pertain to ourselves and our desire for butches."
For information, contact:
grrlburn@earthlink.net

Transmale Mail!

"Got a question? Have experiences to share? Just need to know you're not alone?" Transmale Mail! provides peer support, news, and information of interest to transsexual and transgendered men.
For information, contact: Aaron Davis at
MtMInfo@aol.com or www.onelist.com

Ursula
  For women who identify as bears or with bear
  culture—and their admirers. Ursula is sex-
  positive, inclusive of MTFs and FTMs, butches
  and femmes, and S/M friendly.
  For information, contact:
    kylie@webone.com.au
  To subscribe: visit
    www.webone.com.au/~kylie/ursula.html

Women of Beauty and Temptation
  WomBAT is an e-mail list specifically for
  bisexual women, but any woman may join.
  For information, contact:
    owner-wombat@listserv.aol.com
  To subscribe, send an e-mail to
    listserv@listserv.aol.com
  In the body of the e-mail, type:
    subscribe WomBAT firstname lastname

WHERE TO MEET GIRLS ON THE WEB

Butch-Femme.com
  Free Web personals for butches seeking femmes
  and femmes seeking butches.
  www.butch-femme.com/Romance/personals.htm

Dykesworld Personals
  www.dykesworld.de/Personals/Personals.html

FatGrrl Sex
  Free Web personals.
  www.interlog.com/~miranda/fgs/

GrrlZ on GrrlZ!
  The place to meet women on the Web.
  www.womyn.org/grrlz.html
  us@womyn.org

Lesbian.org
  www.lesbian.org

Muskie's Grrltalk
  The Guide to Lesbian Chat
  A comprehensive overview of lesbian chat
  rooms, with information on how to get started
  with IRC, Web TV, and other live chat
  technology. You can search the site to find chats
  on topics of your choice. Also features personal
  ads and bulletin boards. Says *The Woman's Guide
  to Sex on the Web:* "Ooh, girlfriend! Have you
  ever fantasized about meeting a devastatingly
  competent butch who could show you the ropes
  online? Well, we've got the answer to your
  dreams, and her name is Muskie…"
  www.grrltalk.net/
  muskie@grrltalk.net

Index

About the Author

As publisher of Cleis Press since 1980, Felice Newman has developed and edited books on sexuality and gender by Susie Bright, Joan Nestle, Tristan Taormino, Pat Califia, Carol Queen, Annie Sprinkle, Staci Haines, Loren Cameron, and Cathy Winks and Anne Semans of Good Vibrations. She is a writer and sex educator. She lives in San Francisco.